THE

It can't be measured or monitored or seen on an X ray—but pain can have an undeniable impact on your health and happiness. This important, practical guide explains the facts about chronic pain and provides new hope and help for . . .

- ♦Cancer pain
- ♦Arthritis pain
- ♦Muscular pain
- ♦Back pain
- ♦Headaches
- ♦Carpal tunnel syndrome
- ♦Osteoporosis
- ♦Shingles
- ♦Fibromyalgia
- ♦Postoperative pain
  and other problems

CONQUERING
PAIN

CONQUERING
PAIN

Randall S. Prust, M.D.,
and
Susan Luzader

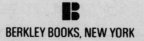

BERKLEY BOOKS, NEW YORK

NOTICE

This book is intended as a reference volume only, not as a medical man-
ual. The information here is designed to help you make informed decisions
about your health. It is not a substitute for any treatment that may have
been prescribed by your doctor. If you suspect that you have a medical
problem, we urge you to seek competent medical help.

CONQUERING PAIN

A Berkley Book / published by arrangement with
the authors

PRINTING HISTORY
Berkley edition / December 1997

All rights reserved.
Copyright © 1997 by Dr. Randall Prust and Susan Luzader.
This book may not be reproduced in whole
or in part, by mimeograph or any other means,
without permission. For information address:
The Berkley Publishing Group, a member of Penguin Putnam Inc.,
200 Madison Avenue, New York, New York 10016.

The Putnam Berkley World Wide Web site address is
http://www.berkley.com

ISBN: 0-425-16118-8

BERKLEY®
Berkley Books are published by The Berkley Publishing Group,
a member of Penguin Putnam Inc.,
200 Madison Avenue, New York, New York 10016.
BERKLEY and the "B" design are trademarks belonging to Berkley
Publishing Corporation.

PRINTED IN THE UNITED STATES OF AMERICA

10 9 8 7 6 5 4 3 2 1

For Justin and Steven

ACKNOWLEDGMENTS

Many thanks to Connie Wicks, R.N., M.S., Barb Lioy, R.N., and Carol Slagel, whose technical and emotional support helped make this book possible. Thanks also to Martha Moutray, who set our feet on the path, and Michele Morris, whose editorial guidance kept us there. We are grateful to the pharmacy staff at Columbia El Dorado Hospital who were always eager to answer our questions, no matter how trivial or complicated. And we will always be grateful to Jerry M. Calkins, M.D., Ph.D., who has filled our lives with truth, fact, and wisdom.

CONTENTS

CONQUERING
PAIN

CHAPTER 1
CONQUERING PAIN

Illness is the doctor to whom we pay most heed; to kindness, to knowledge we make promises only; pain, we obey.

Marcel Proust

EIGHTY PERCENT OF us will suffer from chronic pain some time in our lives. It might be arthritis, it might be cancer, it might be the aftermath of an injury, or it could be shingles, but very few of us will escape. If we're lucky, we'll rest and take a few aspirin or other over-the-counter remedies, and the pain will heal; but for too many, the pain will not go away on its own. It will continue to gnaw at everyday life. Chronic pain, which is pain that lasts longer than it's supposed to, is debilitating to the mind as well as the body, intruding on everything we do.

Pain is universal, crossing all cultural, political, and human boundaries, giving us a basic similarity, but it is a language unique to each of us. There is no technology to measure it, and no matter how many devices or how many techniques we have, pain can only be experienced on an individual level. There is no way to measure how much pain you have. No doctor can put it impartially on a graph or plug your pain into a computer program.

Because it is unique to each and every one of us, it is an individual matter that can't be dealt with like an ailing gallbladder or a broken bone. If your gallbladder is infected, a surgeon removes it. If you have a broken bone, the orthopedist sets it. There are medical schematics to deal with pain, but often an individual's injury or illness takes them off these charts, where the doctor and the patient have to explore various treatments and methods. Pain has a mind of its own, often finding ways around and through normal barriers placed in its way.

But as Bob Dylan says, "The times, they are a changin'." The fear of pain no longer needs to haunt the ill or the injured. By combining techniques, treatments, and medical specialties, health care professionals now have new tools that can lessen or even eradicate chronic pain. Medical science understands pain much better than it did thirty years ago, and understanding leads to solutions.

Just as the general on the battlefield must understand his enemy to develop a game plan, health care providers must know what they are dealing with in order to conquer chronic pain. Technology and recent therapies have given doctors better weapons that go beyond aspirin and bed rest. Spinal cord stimulators, intrathecal pumps, and permanent epidural catheters are some of the big guns in the pain arsenal, but we have learned lots of other ways to help beat pain at its own game.

Knowledge has also taught us that in the pain war, there is strength in numbers. Increasingly, the doctor and the patient are no longer left on their own on the battlefield; they band together with physical therapists, psychologists, nutritionists, chiropractors, acupuncturists, massage therapists, and others as well as physicians from a variety of specialties, to come up with a multipronged attack. A patient with chronic back pain caused by a car accident, for example, might see a neurologist, anesthesiologist, chiropractor, physical therapist, physiatrist (a doctor specializing in physical medicine), acupuncturist, and/or a psychologist. These experts would all communicate on a regular basis, coordinating treatment and prescriptions for the patient, each using the newest techniques in his or her field for the most benefit. Often specially trained nurses help map out and coordinate a comprehensive battle plan.

For example, David, fifty-six, was working as an electrician when a fellow worker opened a door, smashing his arm and shoulder. With a broken thumb, David went to the emergency room where a hand surgeon set the bone. The operation was successful, but for some reason, David developed chronic pain in his arm and shoulder. For most people, the visit to the emergency room and the surgery would result in normal postoperative pain and discomfort for a few weeks, but David had the bad fortune to be one of those few who develop a specific chronic pain syndrome called reflex sympathetic dystrophy (RSD) from his injury. RSD can occur following any trauma, but doctors haven't discovered why some patients develop symptoms while others don't.

David's arm was red, hot, and swollen because of the accident, but instead of the symptoms clearing up as the bone healed, they remained. After a few weeks, the arm became cold, swollen, and painful to any kind of light touch. Just wearing his shirt hurt. In the past, David's arm probably would have been placed in a brace and the wrong type of physical therapy prescribed. This could have resulted in the RSD worsening and David eventually losing the use of his arm.

But because he didn't get better, the surgeon suspected RSD and referred David to a pain center. His first visit confirmed the diagnosis of RSD, so a plan was developed with the surgeon and the physical therapist to stop the cycle of pain so he could return to work. The team employed a combination of nerve blocks, specialized physical therapy, and prescriptions to increase circulation to the arm, as well as creams to desensitize the arm. David went back to work and discontinued all medicines after ten weeks.

You do not have to live with chronic pain. If one doctor or other health care professional can't help you, try another. Pain treatment is an emerging specialty, with professionals banding together to treat this complex and common problem only in the last half of this century. Patients have demanded better pain treatment and we are beginning to deliver it in a more efficient, comprehensive, and compassionate manner. We are learning ways to conquer pain, to fool pain, to short-circuit pain, and improve the quality of life for chronic pain sufferers.

A Brief History of Pain

Until the middle of this century, pain was not generally treated adequately because doctors didn't have the medications or the technology to help the chronic pain patient. The mainstay of the pain arsenal for thousands of years was the opiates derived from the poppy plant. Early writings show that the Greeks, Romans, Chinese, and Egyptians probably used opium plants for pain control, although the Chinese, at least as early as 2600 B.C., also used acupuncture.

The next step in pain control didn't come until the early 1800s when morphine was isolated from crude opium. Then, in 1832, codeine and other opium compounds became available to the public without a prescription, leading to a rash of patent medicines that were said to cure everything from consumption to boils. General anesthesia was first demonstrated to the public in 1846 at Harvard Medical School by W. T. G. Morton, a dentist, although it didn't become widely used until the twentieth century. In the late 1800s, cocaine was used as a local and regional anesthetic.

Sigmund Freud and Carl Jung also experimented with pain control, using psychoanalysis, psychotherapy, and hypnosis to conquer chronic pain, and they met with some success. At about the same time, surgeons began cutting nerves to alleviate pain. And in the middle of this century, doctors developed the technique of using X rays to shrink tumors to reduce pain in cancer patients.

But it wasn't until 1951 that John J. Bonica, M.D., brought the team concept to the treatment of pain, organizing a pain clinic at Tacoma General Hospital in Washington. He brought together physical therapists, surgeons, psychologists, and anesthesiologists to work with chronic pain patients. In 1953, he published *The Management of Pain*, which is still used by health care professionals as one of the definitive books on pain management.

By the 1960s, Bonica and the handful of other pain clinics in the United States had enough scientific data to show that these clinics worked, and pain treatment began to emerge as a medical specialty. Bonica moved his clinic to the University of Washington in Seattle in 1960, and this clinic is still the prototype for pain centers around the world.

But pain management still had a long way to go toward acceptance in most medical training. When I graduated from medical school in 1982, I had received numerous lectures on obscure tropical diseases that I will probably never see, but none on the management of chronic pain. When Bonica studied common medical texts used by students and physicians, he discovered only 0.6 percent of the pages mentioned chronic pain management.

Traditional Western medicine, though, is finally beginning to acknowledge the need for pain management. After all, the number one reason patients see a doctor is for some kind of pain. Pain fellowships are now offered at many medical schools, where anesthesia residents can study pain management exclusively for at least one year after they've completed their anesthesia training.

As traditional Western medicine has started studying and understanding pain, it also is experimenting with nontraditional methods, such as acupuncture. In my anesthesia residency, for example, I was taught by an acupuncturist who was trained in China. A true multidisciplinary approach to pain management incorporates all kinds of methods. The goal is to help the patient and to use whatever works for that individual.

The team approach provides a forum for Western and nontraditional methods. Acupuncture by itself might not work, but acupuncture combined with physical therapy could possibly lessen or eradicate the pain. The multidisciplinary method opens doors to all kinds of possibilities and combinations.

Today, there are multidisciplinary pain centers throughout the United States that offer patients options in managing their pain. When looking for one, make sure it offers more than one kind of treatment. The best pain centers offer physical therapy; psychological pain management techniques; pain block services; referrals to appropriate treatments, such as chiropractic care, homeopathic medicine, and acupuncture; along with the coordination of all this care with an individualized treatment program. These services aren't necessarily located in the pain center, the center simply functions as the hub of the wheel in the treatment of your pain. These centers also work with your primary health care provider to plan the best course of treatment.

As interest in pain management has grown, so have the number of treatments. We now have ultrasound, pain pumps, nerve blocks, and many other options for pain that weren't available twenty or thirty years ago. These new tools complement the advances in knowledge that have emerged as specialists from different areas now work together to help patients. As pain practitioners meet and talk, they exchange ideas and success stories that might help someone else. Acupuncturists now talk with anesthesiologists, physical therapists with psychiatrists, building on each others' experiences and knowledge.

Just as the treatment of pain has changed over the years, the health insurance industry has been changing rapidly, too. Unfortunately, the two have not always taken the same path. Health maintenance organizations (HMOs) tend to rely on set treatments for certain illnesses, like heart disease or diabetes. But pain treatment often doesn't conform to any set treatment and must be individualized. Also, some types of health care coverage don't allow any pain treatment programs.

Because the HMOs are not set up for that kind of treatment, patients might fall through the cracks in the system, or be left undertreated. Patients who demand treatment and are active in their care are the ones who most often get the treatment they need. Some HMOs and insurance plans are much more flexible than others, though, so you should check with your primary care physician about access to pain treatment.

NOT JUST CHRONIC PAIN

In general, all kinds of pain have been undertreated, including acute pain, such as the pain immediately following surgery. Afraid of drug dependency and serious side effects, doctors frequently undertreat this temporary but intense pain. As many as 75 percent of patients experience unrelieved postoperative pain because their doctors don't give them enough medication, and 57 percent of patients going into surgery report that their biggest fear is the pain after the operation. Recent studies show that those who get adequate pain treatment heal more quickly, reduce their hospital stay, and have fewer complications. Hospital stays for major abdominal operations can be cut in half with adequate and aggressive pain control.

Patty, forty-two, had a hysterectomy and was given a patient-controlled analgesia (PCA) pump, where she controlled the amount of pain medication by pressing a button that administered the medicine intravenously. Her roommate refused to have the pump, afraid of the stigma of giving herself narcotics. Patty was up and walking shortly after her surgery, and she was home the next day. She had some discomfort, but no pain. The roommate was still in the hospital when Patty left, unable to walk because of the pain.

New pain control techniques can also get people back to work faster and increase their productivity. Studies show that people who stay out of work for long periods of time are much less likely to ever get back in the workplace than those who get early pain intervention. Even if the pain is eventually brought under control, these patients, for reasons we don't fully understand, never make it back to work. So it is important that chronic pain control be started as soon as possible.

Cancer pain, too, is undertreated. Patients don't have to die in pain, they can be comfortable. We now have the tools

to conquer cancer pain, but the knowledge is still new, and
health care professionals are learning how to use these latest
methods. Not all towns have doctors trained in these skills,
but there are professionals who can help, and more are
learning all the time.

Cancer causes pain, it sometimes causes a great deal of
pain, and in the past, the doctor's primary weapon was the
heavy use of narcotics. Increasing the dose as the pain increased, the patient was often left incoherent and bedridden,
making the final months hard on the family and patient.
The patient was comfortable, but he was basically in a veg-
etative state. Narcotics block pain, but they have serious
side effects, including disorientation, sleepiness, severe
constipation, personality changes, nausea, and even death
if the dosage is increased too quickly. Today, doctors have
techniques developed in the 1980s, such as epidural and
intrathecal pumps that deliver narcotics when the patient
needs them, keeping the patient comfortable and more alert.
These techniques also reduce the serious side effects caused
by giving narcotics orally or in shot form.

WHICH CAME FIRST?

One of the biggest battles faced by patients with chronic
pain has been to get someone to even *believe* they have
chronic pain. Because pain from an injury, for example,
can exist long after the original injury has healed, it has
been difficult for patients to find a health care professional
that understands why they are having pain and how to deal
with it. Too often, the chronic pain patient has been dis-
missed as being a hypochondriac or depressed or simply
someone who wants attention or doesn't want to go back
to work. Often, patients are told their pain has psychological roots, that there's something wrong with them psychologically, and that's why they have pain.

People don't want to experience pain. Some health care
professionals believe that patients invent pain to express

their need for something else. I won't argue that it never happens, but it is very rare in the chronic pain patients I see. Almost all chronic pain patients were leading normal lives until their illness or injury, and they want nothing more than to get back to their normal lifestyle. They weren't clinically depressed before they had chronic pain, but the ravages of chronic pain can lead to serious depression. Statistics show that in the general population, 14 percent are depressed, but in chronic pain patients, that number shoots to anywhere from 30 to 100 percent, depending on the study. Most are depressed because they have pain; they do not have pain because they are depressed.

Bernie, thirty-eight, worked in the lumber industry and enjoyed hunting and fishing with his wife and son and daughter. One day, as he was unloading a truckload of lumber, he slipped. As he fell, he grabbed at a rope, causing boards to crash down on top of him as he tumbled off the truck. He managed to crawl out from under the pile, but as he stood up, he felt a sharp pain in his lower back. He felt that maybe he could walk it off and tried to continue working, but later that night he went to the hospital with severe back pain. Doctors discovered a herniated disc and Bernie underwent surgery a few days later.

Instead of feeling better after the surgery, Bernie felt worse, so doctors continued testing to make certain nothing else had been damaged in the accident. All the tests were negative, so he underwent physical therapy, chiropractic care, nerve blocks, counseling, and transcutaneous electrical nerve stimulation (TENS), but the pain remained. For four years, nothing helped, and the pain was so bad, he couldn't work and rarely left the house. Bernie described his pain as sharp, stabbing, prickling, burning, constant, and throbbing. Just going to the store became a major outing. His wife went back to work to help support them, and Bernie became so desperate that he started talking about killing himself. They decided to move to a warmer climate to see if that would help his back.

In the new city, Bernie went to a neurosurgeon to see if anything else could be done, but was told surgery was not the answer, and the neurosurgeon referred him to a multi-disciplinary pain center. Bernie had weaned himself off narcotics and muscle relaxants and was only taking pre-scription strength ibuprofen. By this time, Bernie had gained close to ninety pounds from sitting around, watching television, and snacking. Unable to work or play, and with the family facing money problems from the loss of his in-come, he yelled at his wife and children in frustration, even driving them out of the house at one point.

At the pain center, Bernie was diagnosed with failed back syndrome, which meant he still had pain following surgery. A psychologist worked with him on relaxation techniques and he went to an anesthesiologist for nerve blocks. The combination gave him some relief, but not enough to get him back to work. At this point, all conservative therapies had failed to give him any long-term relief, so a spinal cord stimulator was suggested. A spinal cord stimulator uses electricity to block the pain signal. A psychologist evalu-ated Bernie and agreed it would be a good idea and a tem-porary stimulator was implanted.

Bernie reported a 90 percent improvement in his pain after one week, and he'd been able to sleep better and move around more. A permanent stimulator was implanted. At his one-month checkup after the stimulator was implanted, Bernie cried for joy in the doctor's office because he could play with his children again and was planning to start vo-cational rehabilitation. He could never do heavy lifting again, but there were still plenty of jobs open to him. Once the pain disappeared, so did Bernie's depression, and he began living a normal life.

As health care practitioners gather information and study the problem more deeply, they find that most chronic pain patients have a physical basis for their pain. Medicine has made great strides in the last thirty years, and we can now track down the physical reason for the pain. We *know* it exists and can treat it. It isn't the patient's fault that he or she has pain, it is a failing of the body that a combination of medicines and techniques can help. Psychologists and psychiatrists are a vital part of any pain team because they can teach ways to help deal with the pain and the psychological damage done by chronic pain. But treating the cause of the pain is the primary goal of any pain team.

Knowledge is power, and that is especially true in the medical field. If you understand pain and its treatments, you have a much better chance of conquering it. This book is not designed to replace any health care professional, but it will give you the information you need to ask the right questions and find the right treatment for your individual needs. We'll also discuss lifestyle changes that can increase your chances of beating pain, but pain management usually requires more than a few self-help tips. There is help for chronic pain, there is more than hope, but it takes effort on your part as well as a team of pain treatment specialists. If you're willing to work at it, you don't have to live with the pain, you can conquer it.

CHAPTER 2
UNDERSTANDING THE ENEMY

Pain is perfect miserie, the worst
Of evils, and excessive, overturns
All patience.

John Milton

TOUCH A HOT stove, and your fingers immediately pull back. Stub your toe, and your foot retreats from the threat. Pain is the body's early warning system, an unpleasant feeling that says something's not right, one of the body's first lines of defense.

As a result, more pain receptors—the nerves that pick up pain signals and pass them to the brain—lie in areas where the body is most likely to get hurt first, such as the hands, feet, and tongue. Groping in a dark room, hands go out in front, much like a cat's whiskers, and the fingers have to be sensitive to locate something that might be dangerous. Fingers or toes test bathwater—not the knee or the chest—ready to jerk back if it's too hot or cold.

The fingers have more pain receptors than the elbow, which has more pain receptors than the shoulder, the body designing its warning system where it's most likely to pick up danger first. A splinter in the fingertip that causes you to flinch would hardly be noticed if it were in the shoulder or the belly.

This doesn't mean an injured shoulder doesn't hurt as much as an injured finger, but it does mean the body notices pain in the outlying areas more quickly, and more intensely, than it does in parts closer to the trunk. Initially, pain is more intense in fingers, toes, and the tongue. The body also places more pain receptors in the skin than it does in muscle, knowing danger from the outside has to pass the skin barrier first.

Though the organs can't feel pain, each is wrapped in a protective membrane that has lots of pain receptors. That's why doctors can perform surgery on a patient's brain while they're awake. Once they anesthetize the skin, bone, and dura mater, the brain's protective covering, surgeons can work on the brain itself with no pain for the patient.

The peritoneum surrounds the organs in the abdomen, and causes pain when it is stretched. A stomachache is actually a peritoneum-ache, because the stomach itself can't feel pain. The pleura protects the lungs and chest cavity, while the pericardium guards the heart. The body has its own alarm system, set to announce any intrusion loudly and forcefully, so you have to react quickly.

Nerves are the electrical wires of the alarm system, sending messages to and from the brain, which processes the information and directs a response. The brain is the command center, rallying resources to keep the body safe and happy. The brain doesn't always make the best decision, though; perhaps the message is scrambled on its way, or it simply doesn't know the correct response to an injury or illness. Arthritis, for example, creates pain that keeps you from using a joint when you really need to keep moving it to prevent more damage.

Pain doesn't travel directly from the site to the brain, but must pass through relay stations as the message makes its way, like messengers handing off important information to the next runner. For example, a pain in the toe doesn't run up one continuous nerve to the brain, but travels along nerves in the leg to the spinal cord, where it goes through a series of nerve tracks, eventually finding its way to the brain. It may be as simple as five or six stops along the way, to many times that for some pain sources. If there was only one nerve leading from the toe to the brain, any damage to that nerve could cut off all sensation and use of that toe. Having various routes and types of nerves gives the body some options when damage or illness affects them, sometimes allowing nerves to reroute around obstacles.

Some nerves carry pain signals faster than others, and different kinds of pain call for different responses. Touching a hot stove, for example, requires a different reaction than a twinge of arthritis pain, and the body routes the pain signal along different nerves to create the correct response. This makes pain complicated, but it also gives health care practitioners several places where the pain signal can be modified or stopped.

Where you hurt may not even be the source of your pain. Your big toe, for example, might be hurting because a nerve coming out from the spinal cord is being pinched, but the nerve goes to the big toe and registers the pain there. This type of pain is called referred pain, because the pain is referred to another area of the body that might be far away from where the damage has occurred.

Because the body doesn't always feel pain where it begins, finding the source of the pain can be complicated. If you have a painful ear, for example, doctors would treat the ear first, checking for infections or something else wrong in and around the ear. But some of the nerves that supply the ear come from the neck, so the source of the ear pain could be a pinched nerve in the neck.

This alarm system is set differently in some people than in others. Doctors can try to grade pain, but they can't really know what the patient is experiencing, relying on the patient to adequately describe the feeling. That is why it is very important to be honest and precise with your health care practitioner when describing pain. Is it sharp? Is it achy? Is it burning? If it feels like a hot poker in your back, then say so. The more information the doctor has, the more he can try to understand your pain.

There are certainly individual variations in pain tolerance, which make people respond differently to the same disease or injury. One appendectomy patient might stay in bed for days, while another is up and around the same day with little or no pain. Some people focus on their pain and it becomes consuming, while others focus outward. These individual differences are what makes pain so unique, and why it is so important to tell your health care practitioner exactly what and how you're feeling.

NOT ALL PAIN IS BAD

Pain can be classified into two broad categories: useful and nonuseful. When someone breaks a leg, they are having useful pain as the early warning system shifts into high gear. That pain is telling them not to use the leg and to get some help. Without pain, the patient would hobble around, making the injury worse. After a reasonable healing period of six to eight weeks, if the patient still has pain, then it's time to reevaluate the injury. The pain could signal an infection or a bone that hasn't healed properly, another example of useful pain.

Herman, sixty, fell in the bathtub, injuring his shoulder. When he first fell, Herman went to the emergency room where an exam and X rays showed no broken bones or other serious injury. Herman was having useful pain, pain that told him to rest his shoulder and seek treatment, and he really didn't need chronic pain management. Instead, he was sent to physical therapy to help with the acute pain and to help the shoulder heal properly. He also took over-the-counter nonsteroidal anti-inflammatory drugs (NSAIDs), such as ibuprofen or naproxen, and was told to apply heat or cold packs, depending on what made him feel better. His shoulder healed in a few weeks with no further problems.

Just because pain is useful doesn't mean it shouldn't be treated, however. Pain after surgery is useful, announcing something has cut into the body, but that doesn't mean the patient should lie in agony while he heals. Pain from a broken bone tells the patient something is seriously wrong, but he shouldn't have to be in pain the six to eight weeks it takes for the bone to knit. While the body uses pain to signal it needs help, that signal should be stopped once the message has been received.

Nonuseful pain has no such noble purpose. Like a car

alarm that keeps shrieking even when the owner returns, nonuseful pain is the early warning system stuck, still irritating, even though it is no longer needed. Nonuseful pain remains long after the initial injury has healed. At one point, it was useful pain, but now it is doing more harm than good, crippling the body it is supposed to protect.

Some pain does no good at all. Arthritis is a classic example of nonuseful pain that is actually detrimental. The pain keeps the patient from using the joint, which actually needs to keep moving to prevent further deterioration. Doctors don't know why nonuseful pain keeps going, but they do know that it can make things worse because the patient often quits using the limb or joint, when using it might actually help the healing process. By not using the area, muscles can atrophy and blood supply can decrease, making the problem worse.

One of the major responsibilities of any pain center is to determine if pain is useful or nonuseful, because the two types are treated differently. Useful pain signals something is wrong, like an infection, illness, or injury. In that case, the source of the pain has to be found and treated, eliminating pain in most cases once the area has healed. Healing the cause stops the pain.

If the pain doesn't stop, then it becomes nonuseful pain, and the chronic pain arsenal can be deployed, turning off the irritating siren. Shingles causes useful pain when it first erupts, letting you and your doctor know the virus has surfaced. Even after the rash and blisters disappear, though, you can be left with debilitating pain that serves no useful purpose.

In addition to determining if pain is useful or nonuseful, doctors must also categorize the pain in order to treat it properly. Pain can be broken down into four types: nerve pain, bone pain, muscle pain, and central pain. All of these types of pain can be useful or nonuseful. Based on the way a patient describes pain, the health care practitioner has to play detective and figure out the source. Treatments vary according to the type of pain, with some better for bone

pain, others for muscle, and still others work best for nerve
pain.

NERVE PAIN

In the strictest sense, all pain is nerve pain. Without nerves
to transmit the pain, you would never feel it. However,
when pain is classified as nerve pain it means the pain originates in the nerve endings, with something pressing on the
area, cutting into it, or otherwise injuring the nerves. An
example would be a herniated disc, where a disc in the
spine slips, pinching a nerve or a group of nerves.

Nerve pain is a very specific type of pain, usually following the path of the nerve, leaving a trail for the health
care practitioner to trace. If a rib nerve is injured, for example, the pain would begin in the rib and could even follow the nerve as it goes into the spinal cord. Because nerve
pain is more predictable, it is generally easier to diagnose
and there are more medical tests to help identify it.

Electromyograms (EMGs) and nerve conduction velocities (NCVs) measure how the muscles respond to stimulation and how well nerves conduct electrical signals, giving
doctors a physical clue to the source. EMGs use a needle
that is inserted into a muscle, sending signals back to a
machine that measures how the muscle responds. Too much
or too little electrical activity lets the doctor know nerves
aren't responding normally to stimulation. By analyzing results, doctors can often determine if the nerve damage is in
the nerve root, the spinal cord, in the muscle, or in a specific nerve or group of nerves. This test is done on an outpatient basis and is uncomfortable, but doesn't usually
require sedation.

NCVs measure how fast a signal travels, because inflammation slows it down. The nerve receives a jolt of electricity to determine if it is conducting signals or if the signal
is disrupted somewhere along the way. Pads are placed
along the nerve, sending small bursts of electricity through

it. By measuring the speed and strength of the signal from one pad to the other, doctors can often determine how and where the nerve is damaged. This test helps determine if specific areas of nerves conduct an electrical signal in a normal way.

These tests also help determine the cause of nerve pain so appropriate treatment can begin. Diabetes causes nerve damage slowly and is treated one way, while a compressed nerve or herniated disc do their damage rapidly and are treated differently. Neither the EMG or the NCV is totally accurate, and they sometimes don't pick up subtle nerve damage.

Typical causes for nerve pain include diabetes, herniated discs in the spine, sciatica, a crush injury, and carpal tunnel syndrome. Patients usually report nerve pain as sharp, traveling, aching, deep, numb, and tingling.

BONE PAIN

Looking at the hard, dry bones on a human skeleton, it doesn't look as if there could be much pain associated with these strong supporters of human bodies. For many years, doctors didn't think bones had any nerves. It was thought all pain originated from the protective membranes, called the periosteum, surrounding each bone. The periosteum has nerves that feel touch, temperature, and stretching. It is a protective layer covering the entire skeletal system, as if it were the skin of the bones. Like the skin, it alerts the nervous system when something attempts to breach the barrier, and that alarm system is pain.

However, scientists have recently discovered tiny nerves do penetrate the bone, so we now know pain can originate directly in the bone itself. The most common type of bone pain is osteoarthritis, or degenerative joint disease (DJD). Everyone develops arthritis as the joints wear out. Ninety percent of people develop some kind by the time they're forty, the disease having started with microscopic lesions in the cartilage by the time they reached twenty.

Even though everyone gets arthritis at some point, it is a mysterious process because the pain serves no useful purpose, perpetuating itself when common sense says the inflammation should have stopped. If you bruise a muscle, the injury heals and the inflammation stops. But with arthritis, the pain continues for no useful reason. Actually, arthritis pain is detrimental because it cripples the body and slows it down, draining energy from other parts.

Diseases that attack the bone also cause bone pain. One of the most common is osteoporosis, a wasting away of the bone mass, weakening it, and possibly causing the bone to collapse on itself (a compression fracture). Osteoporosis is more common in postmenopausal women but occurs in older men, too.

Cancer can invade the bone, causing pain. Breaks and cracks in bones can leave pain behind once they heal, and the same is true with infections. The injuries and infections can damage nerves, which continue to send pain signals after the problem has healed. Anything that decreases blood supply to the bone can cause pain because bones need nutrients supplied by blood, and if that supply is lessened, the bone signals it with pain. Medications, illness, and damage to nerves can keep a healthy supply of blood from getting to the bone, causing pain.

Bone scans are the best test available to detect the origin of bone pain. Radioactive dye is injected into the veins, and the bones absorb the dye, showing defects on an X ray. Healthy bone absorbs the dye differently than abnormal bone, showing where the problem is, but not necessarily what the problem is. This test isn't painful, but it takes several hours for the bones to absorb the dye, so it can take a long time to complete.

Osteoporosis, where the bone isn't as hard as normal bone, can be detected with regular X rays, but doctors often use bone density X rays to determine the severity. Like bone scans, dye is injected into veins where it is absorbed by the bones, giving doctors a clearer idea of the extent of the disease.

Patients usually describe bone pain as deep, aching, and dull, with sharp pain occurring with movement. Even though the pain tends to get worse with movement, it doesn't necessarily go away with rest. The pain is often very specific, staying in one spot.

MUSCLE PAIN

Muscles contain two types of nerves: sensory and motor. The sensory nerves allow the body to feel what is happening to the muscle, and motor nerves put the muscle in motion, coordinating movement, so you can pick up a fork or smile or run a marathon.

The body has three types of muscles: skeletal, smooth, and cardiac. Cardiac does just what it sounds like, controlling the heart. Smooth muscle has no sensory nerves and controls movement of the organs and inner systems, making sure the intestines send food along, the blood vessels send the right amount of blood, and the gallbladder releases digestive fluids—all functions that you don't usually consciously control, called involuntary actions. Skeletal muscle moves the limbs and body, allowing you to squint, snap your fingers, or swim—actions that are generally voluntary, that is, you control them.

When doctors talk about muscle pain, they are usually referring to the approximately 600 skeletal muscles. Cardiac pain is always useful and should be addressed immediately. Smooth muscles can cause pain by not doing their job properly, but they have no sensory nerves, so they can't feel pain.

Certain skeletal muscles contain more nerves than others, especially the hand, feet, and face areas, again, where the body tries to protect itself first. Muscle is the second line of defense for the body, with skin the first, and the nerves are designed to warn the body of danger before it gets deeper. Healthy muscle offers better protection, so it is important to exercise regularly and eat a balanced diet to keep muscles in top shape. Healthy muscles resist strains and sprains better than unhealthy ones, retaining their shape and resilience.

Each muscle is covered by a thin layer of connective tissue containing most of the muscle nerves that feel pain. Usually when you hurt a muscle, the pain is felt most in this protective covering. Stretching or tearing the protective layer causes pain, telling the body to stop whatever it's doing (exercising, stretching, lifting, etc.) before more damage can occur.

Muscles need lots of blood because blood carries oxygen to the muscles and carries away waste products generated by movement. When something slows blood flow to muscles, they hurt, letting you know they need a stronger blood supply. Diseases and injuries to blood vessels, such as diabetes, obesity, and crush injuries, can decrease blood supply. Not using muscles enough also slows blood flow to the area because if you aren't using certain muscles, the body directs blood to other areas where it thinks it's needed more. That's why it's important to stretch lightly before exercising to increase blood flow, preparing the muscle for a workout.

Skeletal muscles are broken down into microscopic parts that allow just a portion of a muscle to move. For example, you need the entire bicep, the muscle that runs from the elbow to the shoulder, to throw a baseball, but you only need a part of it to write a letter. Some of the microscopic parts may be injured, or the entire muscle might be hurt. So muscle pain can mean the entire muscle hurts or it can mean that just a specific part of a muscle is causing pain.

Muscles need to stretch and flex to move the body, but if they are stretched too far, they hurt. Stretching a muscle too much is one of the most common causes of chronic muscle pain. Muscle pain might also be tendon pain. Tendons connect muscles to bones and can be stretched too much or used too much just like muscles. Tennis elbow, where the tendons in the elbow become inflamed from repetitive use, is a classic case of tendon pain. Treatment for tendon pain is usually similar to treating muscle pain.

Muscle pain is usually acute, or useful, pain, and it heals on its own. Strains and sprains are classic examples of muscle pain that hurt a lot at first but eventually heal. Sometimes, though, after the injury heals, the pain remains. Doctors don't know exactly why, but sometimes the injured muscle continues to spasm, depriving the area of oxygen and other nutrients it needs to heal.

Muscle pain is usually described as deep, aching, and dull, with movement making the pain worse. Resting tends to make the pain better, but even during rest, muscles can twitch and move and still cause pain. Unlike nerve or bone pain, patients can sometimes actually see muscle pain as a muscle moves or knots. Unfortunately, medical science hasn't come up with any really good objective tests to detect muscle pain or to even let your doctor know that you have muscle pain.

CENTRAL PAIN

A fourth type of pain, called central pain, originates in the central nervous system, which includes the brain and the spinal cord and causes pain somewhere in the body. Diseases and injuries in the central nervous system can injure nerves in the brain. These injured nerves emit pain signals that the brain interprets as pain in your foot, for example. The central nervous system is confused and thinks the pain is there, when it isn't, it's in the injured part of the brain. A stroke victim, for example, might report a pain in the foot, even though no damage has been done to the foot, and the pain is in fact caused by a damaged brain. Parkinson's disease, multiple sclerosis, and other diseases of the nervous system can also cause central pain.

When doctors can't find an anatomical reason for pain, and other causes have been ruled out, then it's classified as central pain. One way to tell if the pain originates deep within the brain is for the doctor to anesthetize the affected area. If the patient still has pain when all nerves to the area are numbed, then it is probably central pain.

The multidisciplinary approach to pain management as described in chapter 1 is especially important with central pain, because health care practitioners have to rule out any other physical cause for the pain before they can treat symptoms originating in the brain. With all the tests available today, doctors have gotten much better at correctly diagnosing pain so appropriate treatment can begin.

PSYCHOSOMATIC PAIN

There is a difference between pain that begins in the brain and pain that is psychosomatic—pain that feels real but is caused by emotional or psychological factors. Some patients have emotional and psychological problems and it's their mind that needs treatment, not the body. This type of pain benefits from the multidisciplinary approach to pain management, emphasizing psychological and psychiatric help. The multidisciplinary approach helps rule out a physical basis for pain, and can steer the patient toward the kind of help that will benefit them the most.

Your pain is unique; no one else feels what you feel. Because it is unique, treatment must be individualized, adjusted to your level of pain and the reason for it. Your health care practitioner, using tests, a thorough history of your medical problems and pain, and physical examinations has to decide why you have pain before treatment can begin.

Pain alerts you and your doctor to problems that could go unnoticed if the pain didn't act as an early warning signal. But pain can linger even after the problem has healed, leaving you with nonuseful pain that has outlived its purpose. Chronic, or nonuseful, pain lingers long after it is needed, wearing down the body instead of helping it, and exhausting the mind. All pain should be treated, but it is especially important that chronic pain be stopped because it truly does more harm than good.

Whether pain is useful or nonuseful, it needs to be treated and treated aggressively. Don't resign yourself to living with pain. You don't have to. Specially trained doctors and special clinics exist to conquer pain and to give you back a normal life.

In the following chapters, we'll describe some of the more common types of chronic pain, outlining what you and your doctor can do to relieve the pain. You deserve help for your pain, and medical science today has the tools to conquer it.

CHAPTER 3
LOW BACK PAIN

If you believe in evolution, you can trace all of our lower back problems to the time when the first hominid stood erect. If you're a creationist, you can look at it this way: When Eve offered Adam the apple, he stood up to accept it.

Hugo A. Keim

FIVE PERCENT OF adults in the United States experience low back pain each year, and 60 to 85 percent of all Americans will eventually deal with this problem at some point in their lives. In 1990, low back pain was the second leading reason for doctor visits, and the third most common reason for hospital admissions. Twenty million sick days are lost each year to low back pain, costing the United States six billion dollars annually in temporary disability payments.

Most low back pain patients get better in four weeks with or without treatment, but about a quarter of them develop chronic low back pain that stays after an injury heals. Low back pain can happen at any age, and it is the most common reason for disability in people under forty-five, with women having a slightly higher chance of developing it.

Humans get low back pain because they walk upright, placing too much pressure on the lower five vertebrae (lumbar spine) and sacrum (the tailbone), which were originally designed for an animal walking on four legs. That's why walking in water up to the chest often helps back pain, because it takes a lot of the force of gravity off the spine.

In addition to the lumbar region, the spine consists of the middle twelve vertebrae, called the thoracic spine, and the upper seven, called the cervical spine. Each vertebra is shaped like a human stick figure without the legs. The

round, headlike portion is called the body of the vertebra.
The arms are called the transverse process and protect the
nerves. The spinous process is the bone you feel when you
run your finger down your back, and would be the lower
portion of the stick figure. It doesn't add strength or sta-
bility to the spine, but protects the nerves and spinal cord.
Facet joints hold the vertebrae in place, allowing you to
stretch, bend, twist, and turn. The spinal cord runs through
the middle of the vertebra.

The discs lie between each vertebra, acting as cushions
between the bones. Until about the age of twenty, the discs
have their own blood supply. Once we stop growing, this
blood supply stops. Then the discs get nutrients and water
by absorbing them from surrounding vertebrae. As we get
older, the discs get dehydrated and harder, often shrinking,
which can cause the vertebrae to move closer together. This
is one of the reasons we get shorter as we get older.

The discs have a tough outer membrane and are filled
with a gelatinous material called nucleus pulposus. Imagine
a disc like a tire, with the gelatin filling the space where
the air would be. A herniated disc is like a blown tire, with
the gelatin material leaking out, while a bulging disc is like
a tire with not enough air pressure, spreading out because
it isn't full. Discs separate the vertebrae about three-eighths
of an inch, and the nerve roots come out next to the discs,
so if the spaces between the vertebrae narrows, nerves can
be pinched.

NONSPECIFIC PAIN

Low back pain is often broken down into two types: nonspecific and specific. Nonspecific low back pain is generally
caused by sprains and strains, pain that's housed in the
muscles. Ninety percent of this type of pain gets better in
four weeks on its own as the muscles heal, but that doesn't
mean the pain shouldn't be treated to keep the patient comfortable.

Often called the *overdoer's back*, these muscle strains are caused by doing too much of something, such as riding your bike for twenty miles when you normally don't ride it at all, or painting the outside of the house in one weekend, or moving furniture. The muscles are put through more than they're used to and they rebel with inflammation and soreness. This can also stretch ligaments and inflame facet joints not used to this type of movement.

Sudden twists or snapping also cause nonspecific pain, injuring muscles by moving them too quickly. Car accidents are a classic cause of lower back sprains and strains, the jolting surprising the muscles as much as the driver. Drunk drivers frequently escape injury in accidents because the alcohol in their system relaxes their muscles, but the ones they hit are seldom so lucky. If you see the accident about to happen, muscles tense and the sudden force of the crash snaps the muscle. Even if the impact takes you completely by surprise, your body tries to compensate for the jolt by counterstraining in the opposite direction; as the body is suddenly hurled forward, it tries to pull itself back. Even minor car accidents often cause soreness for at least a few days, as the muscles scramble to compensate for the force of the crash.

Other than a physical exam, there are no tests to detect a muscle sprain or strain, but it's that achy soreness that lets the body know it has been damaged and needs to heal. Although it is tempting to crawl into bed when this happens, studies show that two days of rest are as effective as seven days, and staying inactive any longer can actually do more harm than good. Getting up and moving stimulates blood flow, which stimulates the body's immune system. Injuries cause cells to release toxins, and circulating blood carries the toxins away, bringing fresh oxygen and nutrients to the site, so staying in bed for long periods is detrimental. By staying in bed and not using the muscle, the body decreases blood flow to the muscle at a time when it needs more blood to heal.

Although 90 percent of these muscle strains and sprains heal within four weeks, it can be a long four weeks if

you're in pain, so treatments that keep you up and functioning are probably worth the expense and trouble if you
can't move without them. Chiropractic care, massage, acupuncture, physical therapy, biofeedback, muscle injections,
pain medications, and TENS units (they use a small amount
of electricity to stimulate the muscle) are helpful for some
patients. If you've had this pain before and your treatment
worked, then try that treatment again, or ask your doctor
for suggestions.

Ten percent of patients, though, won't get better in four
weeks, and they need further tests and treatment. There's
no way to predict that 10 percent, but there are some clues.
Overweight patients already have too much pressure on
their lower backs from the extra weight. Think about carrying a fifty-pound pack on your back twenty-four hours a
day, and you'll get an idea of what those extra pounds do
to the body. Smokers and those who don't eat a balanced
diet are also less likely to heal quickly because they starve
the body of oxygen and essential nutrients.

Muscle disorders can also cause back pain. Myofascial
pain usually follows an injury of some kind where the muscles were stressed and can't seem to heal. The muscle stays
tight, preventing blood from flowing normally to the area,
cutting off nutrients and oxygen. These tight muscles also
stretch nerves passing through them, causing pain.

Doctors have been describing fibromyalgia for centuries,
but scientists still don't know what causes it. This disease
causes muscles to ache, as if they've been injured, but for
no known reason. Muscles hurt all the time, but no source
for the pain can be found. Chapter 10 contains more information on fibromyalgia.

SPECIFIC BACK PAIN

When a doctor can identify a specific cause for low back
pain, that's specific pain—pain that can be determined by
tests and physical examinations. There are many causes for

specific pain, including an injury or trauma such as a fall or car accident. But it doesn't take a major injury to damage the spine. It could be as simple as making the wrong move at the wrong time. Other causes for specific pain include arthritis, infection, cancer, osteoporosis, compression fracture (where weakened bone is broken from normal stresses), scoliosis (where the spine is curved abnormally), a herniated disc, or spinal stenosis (where the opening for a nerve is too small, pinching it). Imbalances in the body's electrolyte system can also cause pain. The body needs minerals, like potassium, calcium, magnesium, and sodium, to work correctly, and too much or too little cause pain. Taking large doses of over-the-counter minerals could be as harmful as not having enough, and since these imbalances can only be determined through blood tests, you need to work with your doctor to maintain these minerals within a specific range.

Virginia, seventy-eight, woke one night with excruciating pain in her back. She was rushed to the emergency room where X rays showed a compression fracture in her lumbar spine. She was given a mild narcotic and told to see the doctor the next day. He determined that osteoporosis had caused the compression fracture, and sent Virginia to a multidisciplinary pain center for treatment. Because of her age and the type of fracture, the doctor decided against any surgical treatment.

Virginia had been taking the drug warfarin (Coumadin), a blood thinner, that wouldn't allow her blood to clot, so the anesthesiologist at the pain center couldn't perform an epidural because of danger of blood getting into the epidural space. An epidural uses a needle to inject some local anesthetic and steroids into the space between the ligaments of the spine and the nerve, called the epidural space. She was given trigger point injections, where a local anesthetic is injected into the muscles to relax them, as a temporary measure. Virginia was given a TENS (transcutaneous electrical nerve stimulator) unit, which delivers a small electrical current to the muscles through pads on the skin, helping to block the pain signal.

Working with her cardiologist and her primary care doctor, the warfarin was stopped so the anesthesiologist could try an epidural. When her blood clotting returned to normal, the doctor performed a lumbar steroid epidural, which means some steroids and local anesthetic were injected into the lumbar (lower back) portion of the epidural space. Compression fractures cause inflammation in the nerve roots, the epidural space, and the area around it, including the muscles. The inflammation causes pain, and the goal of the epidural is to reduce the inflammation, allowing the area to heal.

Virginia had some relief, and she was told to apply capsaicin cream to the painful area. A few days later, she was given a second epidural, the pain became 30 percent better, and she quit using the TENS unit. She found it hard to apply capsaicin cream to her back, so she quit using it. The third epidural allowed her to quit using narcotics for the pain, and she was able to walk around and sleep better. Her primary care doctor put her on medication for osteoporosis, and she returned to her normal lifestyle.

Carlos, thirty-six, was an airline baggage handler who twisted his back while lifting a heavy bag. He went to a chiropractor for eight months and the pain was much better, but then he reinjured his back and the chiropractic care quit working. He went to an occupational medicine specialist who prescribed over-the-counter pain medications and put him in a back strengthening program. After four weeks, Carlos reported his pain was a five to eight on a scale of ten, with ten being the worst pain he could imagine, and the low back pain had spread to his groin and right leg.

Carlos was referred to a neurosurgeon who ordered an MRI (magnetic resonance imaging, which gives a picture of the inside of the body using magnetic frequencies). The MRI showed a small herniated disc. The neurosurgeon thought the herniated disc looked too small to be causing all the pain and the surgeon referred Carlos to a multidisciplinary pain center.

At the pain center, the doctors agreed the disc wasn't compressing any nerves and discovered the pain was caused by an injured sacroiliac joint, which lies between the tail-bone and the pelvis. He was sent to a psychologist who taught him biofeedback and other techniques to manage the pain. An anesthesiologist gave him injections in his muscles and joints to relieve the pain and inflammation so he could undergo more physical therapy.

Within four weeks, after undergoing three series of injections, three sessions with the psychologist, and twelve rounds of physical therapy, Carlos's pain was down to a two out of ten, and he went back to work. Because of the small herniated disc, though, he was restricted to light duty and eventually found a job repairing airplanes.

What You Can Do

Paying attention to the pain is the patient's most important job. A major car accident, a fall from a stool or ladder, or any minor injury in an older person or one with osteoporosis should be checked immediately by a doctor. You should also see a doctor if you have any of the warning signs of back pain, which signal that your pain needs treatment right away. Night pain that's waking you up, pain that worsens when you lie down, weakness in your legs, trouble controlling your bowels or bladder, trouble walking, loss of strength in legs and feet, numbness or tingling in legs, and a fever or chills are all symptoms that should send you immediately to the doctor.

Also, people over fifty years old and those under twenty should be especially careful. Once we're past fifty, the body begins wearing out and even minor trauma can cause serious injury. Those who are under twenty years old usually don't complain much and can let potentially serious injuries slide for too long, so if a person under twenty has been in an accident and complains, those complaints should be addressed right away.

If you have none of the warning signs, it is still important to see a doctor if the pain is keeping you from working or enjoying a normal lifestyle. If you've sprained your back before and recognize the symptoms, then try whatever worked before. However, do not use any leftover prescription medication from a previous injury without first asking your doctor, and never let anyone talk you into trying some prescription that their doctor gave them. Medicines react differently with different people, and they can interact with something you're already taking, so always check with your doctor or pharmacist before mixing medicines.

Most patients start with heat or ice packs and over-the-counter pain medications. Heat increases blood supply to the area, while cold decreases the blood supply. Cold penetrates deeper than heat and reduces inflammation, so cold packs may be more effective for sprains and strains. Never place ice directly on the skin because it can cause frostbite. Wrap the ice or cold pack in a towel or other thick cloth and never leave it on the area for more than fifteen minutes, unless your doctor tells you to.

After two to three days, when the inflammation subsides, then heat can bring more blood to the injured muscle, carrying away toxins and bringing nutrients. As with ice, heat should never be applied directly to the skin, and if the skin becomes bright red, take the heat source away. A heating pad is usually a safe way to get heat to injured muscles because it regulates the heat, not letting it get too hot. If you have swelling, it's a good idea to use ice packs, but once the swelling goes away, then heat may be the best choice. When there's no obvious swelling, use heat or ice, whichever makes the area feel best.

Always carefully read the warning labels on over-the-counter medicines, and ask your pharmacist for advice and suggestions if you have any questions. Generally, avoid bed rest, or if you absolutely have to, limit it to two days. Keep moving, but use good body mechanics. Don't twist your back or bend from the waist, stand and sit straight because slumping puts more pressure on the back and pulls it out of alignment. And avoid any movement that causes the pain to increase.

In the first four weeks, if you don't have any of the warning signs, look for techniques and treatments that might relieve your symptoms. Studies show chiropractic care relieves pain for some people. Acupuncture, acupressure, and massage also work for some patients, although the scientific proof is lacking. Pool exercise, usually beginning two weeks after the initial injury, can be very beneficial because it takes weight off the injured back, allowing you to condition it without stress. Walking is another good exercise for back pain.

Over-the-counter liniments or creams that you rub on the sore area help some patients, and each have slightly different ingredients. Ask your pharmacist for advice on which ones to use for your type of pain, or ask friends about what worked for them. Some of the creams contain capsaicin, which is derived from chili peppers, so be sure to wash your hands thoroughly after using them or wear rubber gloves when applying the cream. If you accidentally rub your eyes while the cream is still on your hands, it will burn, but will not do any permanent damage. Capsaicin can also cause the skin to burn. If this happens and it becomes too uncomfortable, soak a paper towel in milk and apply it to the burning area.

Back supports, sometimes called lumbar supports, are those wide belts fastened with Velcro worn by some workers who do a lot of lifting, and they sometimes relieve lower back pain. You don't need a prescription for these, and can buy them in drug stores and other places that sell medical supplies. Back braces are fitted individually and are made of plastic or metal to support the back like an extra bone or muscle. They must be prescribed by a doctor and used with supervision because they can do more harm than good.

Devices sold through television or magazine ads tempt many people suffering from pain. Sometimes they'll work on your pain, but remember, 90 percent of patients get better in four weeks with or without treatment, and you need to evaluate what exactly these "cures" are offering. Some send small amounts of electrical current to injured muscles, while others stretch or massage muscles. Try less expensive methods first, such as exercise and over-the-counter medi-

cations, before paying for fancy devices that probably
won't work.

Where you sleep can also affect the health of your back.
When you sleep, the muscles in the back relax and can be
pulled in ways that wouldn't happen when awake. An old,
soft mattress with lumps and bumps can pull the back out
of alignment, putting more pressure on one side than another, making back pain worse. If your back pain is worse
in the mornings, then take a careful look at your mattress.
If you think it's too soft, try putting a board between the
mattress and box spring, or try sleeping on the floor for a
night or two to see if it helps. If you decide to buy a new
mattress, make certain it has a guarantee that you can
exchange it after a few weeks if it isn't working for you.
You may have to try several before finding the right one.
The early versions of water beds didn't give enough support
for the back and the waves put extra stress on the muscles,
but modern ones with individual chambers filled with water
do a much better job of supporting the back.

Maintaining good health is one of the most important
things you can do to help your back heal. By keeping your
weight in the normal range, you keep excess force off the
bones and discs and reduce the risk of injuring your back
again. A diet with lots of fresh vegetables and fruits and
whole grains not only helps you maintain a healthy weight,
but also gives your body the nutrients essential for healing.
Magnesium and calcium supplements can help tight muscles relax, reducing spasms.

Avoid substances that reduce blood flow to the injured
area. Caffeine constricts blood vessels, clamping them
down when the muscle needs all the flow it can get to wash
away toxins. Nicotine has the same effect, starving the injured area of nutrients, while not allowing harmful substances to be washed away. Alcohol depresses the immune
system, keeping it from healing properly, and also prevents
the body from absorbing essential nutrients. Alcohol is a
poison that kills cells just when the body needs new ones
for the healing process, and it damages nerves, which need
to be in top shape if you ever expect to get rid of the pain.

All of the above treatments can work for both specific and nonspecific pain. If your doctor diagnoses specific back pain, though, you'll have to decide if you want to take aggressive action right away, such as surgery, or if you want a more conservative approach, such as physical therapy and pain blocks. Before you make any decisions, though, you want to make certain you have as much information as possible.

Ask your doctor to explain his findings completely and then present you with alternatives. Don't be afraid to get more than one opinion, and don't be afraid to ask questions until you understand what is wrong and what are the possible solutions.

If you decide on surgery, ask your surgeon how many of these surgeries he performs each year. Chances are, the doctor who does 100 of these operations a year is going to be more proficient than one that does 10. Ask to speak to other patients who have had the same surgery to find out what you can expect afterward, and be prepared to take time off from work and to attend whatever therapies the doctor prescribes.

In general, there are two types of surgeons who operate on the back. Orthopedic surgeons treat bone injuries and diseases and receive at least five years of training after they graduate from medical school. Neurosurgeons specialize in the nervous system and train six to nine years after graduation from medical school. Orthopedic surgeons will usually fix bones in the back, while neurosurgeons will operate on the spinal cord and discs. If a surgery is complicated, the two might work together. Your primary doctor will help you decide which is right for your problem.

Before you even consider surgery, be certain you have specific back pain and the doctors know exactly what is wrong with you. Never have an operation just because you have pain; you must know what is wrong and what the doctor intends to do to fix it. There are doctors who will operate without knowing the exact cause of the pain, hoping the surgery will somehow help.

What Your Doctor Can Do

After four weeks of persistent pain with none of the warning signs, it's time to see your family doctor. The doctor will examine you and listen to your history, both clues that will lead him toward a diagnosis and treatment. Patients should be prepared to make a time commitment to attend physical therapy and other treatments. Sometimes, one of the most difficult things patients do is to find time to get better.

Your doctor might order a set of X rays, which will pick up problems with bone, such as arthritis, bones out of alignment, cancer, some cases of spinal stenosis, osteoporosis, and compression fractures (where the vertebrae have weakened and the force of gravity breaks them). A bone scan also picks up problems with the vertebrae, and is especially good at finding inflammation. Dye is injected in a vein and an image taken, much like an X ray, showing problem areas in the bone as it absorbs the dye.

Computerized tomography (CT scan), a specialized X ray, is another test for bone defects. Magnetic resonance imaging (MRI) is better at finding problems with soft tissue, such as the discs and nerves. MRIs use a magnetic field to produce a computerized image of the body and require specialized radiologists to read the X rays. CT scans can cost $700 and up, while MRIs cost $1,500 and up. Insurance generally covers the cost of these tests. Some patients think they need an MRI right away, but it may not be the correct test for their pain, especially if the doctor suspects bone damage.

Electromyograms (EMGs) measure how muscles respond to stimulation. The doctor inserts a needle into the muscle and a machine measures how it responds to electrical stimulation. Nerve conduction velocities (NCVs) use pads placed along a nerve that send an electrical signal to see how and where the nerve is damaged. Both these tests are uncomfortable, but they are necessary if the doctor suspects nerve damage because they can pinpoint where and what the damage is.

A doctor might also order blood tests to pick up electrolyte imbalances and blood diseases, such as sickle cell anemia, that might cause back pain. He could order other, more specialized tests, but in general, he will order one or more of the above.

Once he has a diagnosis, the doctor can begin a course of treatment. Your family doctor may be able to treat you, depending on his training and the direction you want your treatment to take. In most cases, nonsurgical options will be tried first, unless there are clear indications for immediate surgery, such as a life-threatening situation, or if the doctors think permanent damage is occurring. A bulging disc, for example, almost never requires surgery, and only 10 percent of patients with herniated discs need immediate surgery.

Often, doctors order a rehabilitative back strengthening program using physical therapy to create stronger back muscles. The physical therapist will teach you exercises you can do at home or at the gym to maintain a healthy back and help prevent future injuries.

Physical therapy can help both specific and nonspecific pain by making room for pinched nerves as it strengthens ligaments, correcting the problem by making the back stronger. Physical therapy also reduces inflammation by stimulating the body's immune system through movement and allowing blood to flow more freely to the injured area.

In addition to exercise, therapists might use ultrasound, which sends energy waves to the affected area, increasing blood flow. Massage, as well as hot and cold packs, can be used, and microcurrents, which send small amounts of electricity to the injured area to increase blood flow may be helpful, although no studies exist to prove they work. Myotherapy (stretching) is another tool of physical therapists.

All these therapies also help muscles in spasm. When a muscle spasms or cramps up, it knots into a ball, slowing blood flow to the center. By smoothing the spasm, the physical therapist can get blood flowing into the area that most needs it.

Physical therapists have specific techniques for individual problems, and will design sessions to fit your needs. It is best to see the same physical therapist every time you go in because he will know your body and its problems. You don't see a different doctor every time you go in, and you shouldn't see a different physical therapist each time.

Manipulation therapy practiced by chiropractors and doctors of osteopathy (DOs), can also be useful. Both physical therapy and manipulation therapy increase blood circulation, allowing the body's healing mechanisms to bring in nutrients and wash away toxins.

After six sessions with the physical therapist, DO, or chiropractor, if you aren't noticing any positive change, then it's time to go back to your family doctor or get a second opinion. A positive change in six sessions may not mean a decrease in pain, although that is the ultimate goal, but you may notice you are able to move better or have more strength, signs that the sessions are beginning to work.

Your doctor may also put you on medication to relieve inflammation and pain. The most common type of analgesics for low back pain are nonsteroidal anti-inflammatories (NSAIDs), stronger cousins of the ones bought over the counter. The newer prescription NSAIDs tend to have fewer side effects than their earlier counterparts, which sometimes caused problems with the digestive system, liver, and kidneys. These newer drugs only need to be taken once or twice a day instead of three or four times. Always take NSAIDs with a full meal to avoid irritating the stomach.

Muscle relaxants may be prescribed to reduce spasms, and nonnarcotic analgesics can be used to ease pain. Steroids are sometimes prescribed to reduce inflammation, but usually only for short periods of time because they are very potent and have many side effects. Some antiseizure medicines have been found to help with nerve pain, while some antidepressants have been shown to help with some nerve and muscle pain. More information on all the drugs listed above can be found in chapter 11.

Narcotics are also very potent and are prescribed for severe, debilitating pain and are also usually taken for short periods of time. Chapter 12 gives more details on narcotics.

Hypnosis and biofeedback are useful tools to help back pain, teaching the patient to use his mind to battle the effects of the pain.

For especially persistent pain, doctors might try a transcutaneous electrical nerve stimulator (TENS), which uses pads on the skin that deliver small amounts of electricity to block the pain signal.

Muscle stimulators strengthen muscles by delivering electrical current directly to the muscle. Pads are placed over the muscle and an electrical current, which tingles, causes the muscle to contract as if you were using it. This keeps the muscle from wasting away when pain prevents you from using it. By strengthening the muscles, they can support the back better, performing the job they were supposed to do.

Some patients report acupuncture helps with low back pain, although scientists haven't come up with conclusive evidence that it does.

Psychological or psychiatric care is useful for some patients, and is usually used in combination with other therapies. Specially trained psychologists and psychiatrists help patients learn to deal with the pain, and usually only see the patient for a short period of time to teach pain control techniques, such as relaxation, hypnosis, and biofeedback.

Nerve blocks administered by an anesthesiologist may also be prescribed to break the cycle of pain and allow the body to heal itself. The most common nerve block in specific low back pain is a steroid epidural. The steroids used are the same as the ones taken orally, but in a smaller amount, and they are injected in the area between the ligaments of the vertebrae and the spine, called the epidural space, where the nerves are concentrated in a small space before they leave the spine. Injecting steroids helps wash away toxins in the space, something like changing the oil

in a car. The steroids help reduce inflammation, which allows more room for the nerve roots and the spinal cord,
easing pressure that may be causing pain. Most anesthesiologists offer the patient a sedative before an epidural, and
then numb the skin with a local anesthetic before inserting
the needle. It is slightly uncomfortable, but shouldn't hurt.
If it is painful, something probably isn't right. Steroid epidurals are usually limited to no more than three in six
months because the medicine is so powerful.

Muscle, joint, and nerve injections are another treatment
option. The doctor injects a small amount of steroid and
local anesthetic or possibly a small amount of prescription
NSAIDs directly into the muscle, joint, or nerve near the
skin, with deeper nerves requiring more complex injections.

Trigger point injections are used for muscle pain and
spasms. Trigger points are scattered all around the muscles
and are centers for relaying information, like relay stations.
By pressing on these points, the doctor or therapist can
recreate the pain. If pressing on a trigger point recreates the
pain, it can signal that this is at least one point where the
pain may originate. Trigger points often correspond with
acupuncture points, both relay stations for electrical signals.
When muscles tighten from injury or illness, they can irritate these relay stations, causing pain.

Depending on the type of pain and the patient, doctors
will inject a variety of substances into the trigger point to
help the muscle relax, resetting the pain signal, interrupting
it, and turning off the alarm. Sometimes, a dry needle will
be inserted into the trigger point and twisted, other times,
local anesthetic, water, plant enzymes, NSAIDs, or steroids
will be injected.

Lumbar sympathetic nerve injections are usually done in
an outpatient clinic or hospital because the doctor uses an
X ray to guide the needle. These shots use local anesthetic
in a specific nerve or group of sympathetic nerves (the
nerves that control functions you normally don't think
about, like breathing, digestion, and blood circulation), to
increase the blood flow to the painful area. Some patients
need a sedative for these injections, and the skin is numbed

before the needle is inserted, with the numbing medicine continually administered as the needle moves through the body.

Facet joints, which help the spine move, sometimes contract arthritis. Diagnosing and treating this problem involves injecting a local anesthetic and steroids into the arthritic facet joint under X ray.

Occasionally, when all other options have failed, doctors will inject chemicals into a nerve to kill it. Radiofrequency and cryoanalgesia can also be used to kill nerves. They are described in chapter 13. Killing a nerve can cause complications and the nerve almost always grows back, sometimes bringing worse pain when it does.

Deep nerve blocks are done in nerves that are more than an inch below the skin, and they should be done in an outpatient clinic or hospital. A hospital or clinic will have all the equipment necessary to deal with any complications. Some require X rays to help place the needle, and all these injections are more risky because the deeper the needle goes into the body, the greater the risk of hitting something it shouldn't. The needle is inserted and the medicine given quickly, so the pain only lasts a few seconds.

If none of the above therapies are working after trying them for two or three weeks, then you need to talk to your doctor about a multidisciplinary pain clinic. Often, the above treatments work fine by themselves, but when they don't, then it is time to try an individualized program using a combination of techniques. Perhaps nerve blocks would help the physical therapy be more effective, or perhaps the patient needs some psychological tools to help him deal with the pain. Studies show that for chronic pain, the multidisciplinary clinics are more effective than single treatments.

SURGICAL OPTIONS

Surgery may be necessary immediately if the problem is too dangerous to try other methods. Surgery should never be done unless the surgeon has a specific diagnosis, because performing surgery just because the patient has pain almost never works. But just because there's a diagnosis, doesn't mean surgery has to be the first step. Most surgeons use the multidisciplinary approach if surgery isn't necessary immediately, trying other methods before resorting to an operation.

The goal of surgery is to correct a problem. If there's a herniated disc, surgeons take out the herniated part. If the nerves are being compressed by bones, they give the nerves more room. Most back surgeries fall under the broad category of laminectomies, which simply means removing a portion of the lamina on the vertebrae. The lamina connects the head of the vertebra to the transverse process, and sometimes has to be removed to give the surgeon access to the spinal canal, nerve roots, or the disc, where he can correct whatever is causing the pain. Laminectomies might be used to correct herniated discs or spinal stenosis. These surgeries can last as little as an hour, and the patient usually recovers in four to six weeks.

Fusions are another type of back surgery, although not nearly as common as laminectomies. Fusions stabilize a spine that has been damaged by scoliosis, a tumor, or some other disease that erodes the bone. Metal rods or bone grafts are inserted next to the spine to strengthen it, bridging the damaged area. Always get a second opinion from another surgeon before agreeing to this operation because this is a complicated procedure requiring four or more hours of anesthesia and surgery. Recovery time from a fusion can be months or even years.

Erma, thirty-six, began experiencing low back pain for no reason that she could remember, but the pain kept getting worse and began traveling down her legs, especially her right leg. Her doctor ordered X rays, which showed a herniated disc and she was sent to a surgeon who performed a laminectomy and fusion. After surgery, she had occasional pain, but was much better and took medications only for flare-ups.

Four years later, she was pulling back the cover on her

pool when the pain returned, similar to what she'd had before the surgery. She was sent to a neurologist who determined she had some nerve degeneration, but no herniated disc or stenosis (where the spinal opening is too small, pressing the nerves). There was some scar tissue around the nerve roots from the surgery, but nothing that required further surgery.

The neurologist referred Erma to a multidisciplinary pain center where an anesthesiologist felt she had a sprain from pulling back the pool cover, which had aggravated the nerve roots affected by the scar tissue. She was given an epidural and only got a little relief. After the second epidural, though, she was sent to physical therapy, and the pain was reduced significantly to the point where she was back to the level before the pool cover accident and only took medications for occasional flare-up pain.

Erma was like a lot of patients after surgery who have good results, but then injure themselves again. Often, they think they've developed the same problem, when it might be something else, such as irritated scar tissue.

Spinal cord stimulators (SCSs), which use electrodes next to the spinal cord to block the pain signal, are options for patients who can't be helped with surgery. They are used as a last line of defense, and only for patients who have exhausted more conservative therapy. SCSs have a 75 percent success rate when they are used in carefully selected patients.

Intrathecal pumps can be effective initially, but no studies show if they are effective in the long term. They are usually used only after both conservative treatments and SCSs don't work. Pumps and the medicines used in them are steadily improving, increasing the benefits and decreasing the risks. Pumps and SCSs are discussed more in chapter 13.

As with any surgery, there are potential complications from back operations, but with today's technology, they are uncommon. Always make sure you understand the possible risks of an operation and what your chances are for developing them.

FAILED BACK SYNDROME

Failed back syndrome, sometimes called postlaminectomy syndrome, occurs in about 30 percent of back surgery patients. The term tells exactly what happens: the surgery was a success, but the pain remained. In other words, the surgeon can no longer find any reason for the continuing pain. For example, in a laminectomy to repair a herniated disc, the surgeon successfully fixed the disc, but the patient continued to have pain.

If the patient's original pain disappears after the surgery, but a new one appears, it could be scar tissue. Surgeons rarely operate to remove scar tissue that might be causing pain because the second surgery will only cause more scar tissue, so other methods have to be tried. If the original pain remains, then it becomes more difficult to determine what's causing the pain.

Evaluating the patient in a multidisciplinary pain center at this point is usually a good idea, because doctors have to start over again to determine the cause of the pain. These cases are more complicated and require a focused, individualized pain program to find a possible second cause for the pain.

Failed back syndrome sometimes responds to SCSs, and a new type, with dual electrodes, seems to be especially effective for this type of pain.

ARACHNOIDITIS

Spiderwebs of inflammation and scar tissue wrapped around the spinal cord characterize arachnoiditis, a complication of back surgery, trauma, meningitis, or other disease. This condition is especially insidious because even if the inflammation is tamed, the scar tissue remains, tugging on the spinal nerves.

Unlike other types of low back problems, arachnoiditis generally doesn't respond well to physical therapy and other treatments. The scar tissue is inside the spinal canal, where more conservative treatments can't reach it. Surgery is never indicated for this disease because it will only add to the scar tissue, making the problem worse. Usually, the arachnoiditis patient benefits from a multidisciplinary approach because it often takes more than one type of treatment to keep this disease under control.

Low back pain cripples millions of Americans each year, but as medicine learns more about how and why the back functions, and what causes the pain, it also learns ways to help. Although our bodies haven't yet caught up with our ability to walk upright, modern methods and technologies are helping us overcome our natural shortcomings.

CHAPTER 4

REFLEX SYMPATHETIC DYSTROPHY (RSD) OR COMPLEX REGIONAL PAIN SYNDROME (CRPS)

The body never lies.

Martha Graham

THERE IS NO exact figure for the number of people afflicted with reflex sympathetic dystrophy (RSD), but estimates place it in the millions. RSD is the result of an injury. Whether it is something as minor as a bug bite or something as traumatic as a shotgun blast, some outside force disrupts the body's sympathetic nervous system, which regulates the heartbeat, blood pressure, skin temperature, and other body functions that generally work without conscious interference. This disruption confuses the body, and it responds by signaling pain to let you know it feels something is wrong.

Up to 5 percent of nerve injuries lead to RSD, with some of the milder cases healing on their own, but still leaving many with a pain that seems greater than expected from the initial injury. RSD needs to be treated early before the syndrome permanently damages tissue.

Following most injuries, patients experience the normal pain of healing, but RSD exists long after the initial injury heals. Symptoms may begin a few days after the injury or it may take several weeks for RSD to appear. Some of the common symptoms include pain, swelling, skin color changes, hypersensitivity, weakness, wasting away of muscle, limited motion, and reduced skin temperature around the affected area or limb.

The primary clue that a patient has RSD is if he has pain out of proportion to what an examination and tests would indicate. For example, if a jug of milk falls on a patient's foot, he would go to a doctor for X rays to see if it was broken. If there wasn't a break and the pain kept getting worse and worse, instead of slowly healing, he'd go back to the doctor to try to find out why. This is where the RSD patient begins a search for a name to this pain and for a solution.

Keith, age forty, ruptured a disc in his lower back and had surgery to repair it. The pain from his injured back disappeared after the surgery, and he was looking forward to getting better because he and his wife were expecting their first child a month later. He attended physical and rehabilitation therapy, and his recovery progressed normally.

After a week, though, Keith developed a new pain in his right leg, unlike any he had before the surgery. His leg became sensitive to touch, so that even sheets covering his legs kept him awake at night. The leg ached and burned, swelled, and felt sometimes hot, and sometimes cold. His surgeon worried about possible infection from the surgery, but an examination disproved that theory.

The surgeon then suspected RSD and sent Keith to a multidisciplinary pain center where doctors confirmed RSD. He was given a series of three nerve blocks along with physical therapy and doctors prescribed antidepressants and gabapentin, an antiseizure medicine that helps with RSD. Keith improved, but once the blocks ceased, his pain returned.

An anesthesiologist recommended a continuos epidural (local anesthetic and narcotic pumped into the epidural space) for one week with intensive physical therapy. His insurance company wanted a second opinion, and Keith was given trigger point injections by another physician, but these weren't successful and the pain became worse, so he returned for the epidural.

After a week, the epidural was removed and he could return to his job and normal activities, including playing with his new daughter.

NERVOUS SYSTEM GONE AWRY

RSD frustrates both the patient and health care professionals. The only symptom shared by all patients afflicted with RSD is pain, which makes early diagnosis and treatment difficult. RSD symptoms and signs have been documented since the 1500s, but because symptoms vary from person to person, doctors still have trouble today identifying this tricky syndrome. There is no recognized objective medical test for RSD, and it usually has to be diagnosed primarily by a thorough patient history and physical examination. There are tests that can help diagnose RSD, but they aren't definitive, and sometimes someone who has RSD might have a negative result on those tests. Diagnosis is even more complicated because some health care professionals don't believe it exists.

Controversy surrounds even the naming of this group of symptoms, which can add to the patient's confusion. There is a trend toward naming this group sympathetically mediated pain syndromes (SMPS) or complex regional pain syndrome (CRPS), but RSD is a more common name and one health care professionals are more likely to use for now.

To make it even more complicated, RSD is an umbrella term that covers several types of pain. There are many names for specific types of RSD, such as shoulder-hand syndrome, minor causalgia (an injury to a nerve involving bullets or shrapnel), and posttraumatic pain syndrome.

Although scientists learn more about RSD all the time, health care professionals still don't know why an injury triggers this painful syndrome, and they don't know why it affects some people and not others. It's also a mystery why the nervous system in the RSD patient does the opposite of what it should do for an injured area. Normally, the body would want to increase blood flow to an injury, sending oxygen and other nutrients to speed healing, but in RSD, the blood vessels clamp down, turning the area cold and purple.

In the early stages of RSD, the body *does* send too much blood to the injury, and then the veins don't carry away all that blood being pumped into them, causing a red, hot, swollen, painful limb. The limb turns red and swells because the veins are not carrying away the excess blood and the arteries continue to pump blood, building pressure in the area. These are early signs of RSD, but they can also be signs of infection and other complications of an injury, thus making RSD difficult to diagnose at this early stage.

Dennis, fifty-one, hurt his right wrist on the job. He was treated by an occupational medicine physician who took X rays, put him in a wrist splint, and gave him some nonsteroidal anti-inflammatories (NSAIDs). In most patients, this would have been enough to allow the injury to heal, but Dennis developed RSD in his arm, which became cold, swollen, and painful.

He attempted to go back to work but couldn't do his job because of the pain, which caused him to have limited motion in his right arm. His occupational medicine doctor was reluctant to prescribe narcotics for the pain because Dennis was a recovering alcoholic. Alcoholics tend to have an addictive personality, so supplying them with narcotics may be too much of a temptation, and alternative treatments are needed. Dennis returned to work, taking prescription nonsteroidal anti-inflammatories for the pain.

Dennis returned to the doctor several months later because he was still in pain, but the doctor couldn't find a reason for the pain, so Dennis was referred to a multidisciplinary pain center. Dennis's right arm was swollen, weak, cold, hypersensitive, and had a splotchy purple color. In this case, because he had many of the classic RSD symptoms, Dennis was diagnosed fairly quickly.

While the pain center waited for his insurance to approve a course of treatment, Dennis was placed on calcium channel blockers and tricyclic antidepressants. Calcium channel blockers open small blood vessels to allow increased circulation to the area, and the antidepressants reduced the pain so he could sleep better, but in Dennis's case, the medicines weren't effective enough. Dennis was still not able to work, even with this drug therapy, so the pain center moved to the next step.

Dennis's sympathetic nervous system was clamping down on the blood vessels in his arm, decreasing blood flow to the area. He was given nerve blocks, allowing the blood vessels in his arm to increase blood flow, followed with intense physical therapy. Physical therapy in RSD patients is usually too painful unless nerve blocks are given first, but sometimes patients are able to tolerate physical therapy without blocks, especially in early, mild cases of RSD. In some patients, nerve blocks alone work, and in others, physical therapy is enough to stop the pain, but in general, a combination of the two gives the best chance for recovery.

Dennis was given a series of nerve blocks, along with the physical therapy, for eight weeks. After the treatments, he was 80 percent better and he returned to work, where he continued to improve.

THREE STAGES

There are three stages to RSD: the early stage, the dystrophic stage, and the late (atrophic) stage. There is a much higher treatment success rate if RSD is caught in the first stage, before the decreased blood supply causes a permanent loss of function in the arm, leg, or other area. If RSD is caught at this early stage, the success rate is very high. In both the early and dystrophic stages, doctors can actually cure RSD, but cures are rare when it reaches the atrophic stage. They can treat the pain in this late stage, but can't undo the damage.

In the early stage, the symptoms tend to be in the area around the initial injury. This stage might last only a few days or stretch into months and is characterized by a red, hot, tender, and swollen area where too much blood is being pumped to the site and not enough carried away.

One major symptom of RSD, even at this early stage, is a hypersensitivity around the injury. With a broken bone, for example, the patient has the normal pain of the injury, but with RSD, the skin over the broken bone is so sore that just touching it causes severe pain. With a broken wrist, most patients can move it somewhat, but with RSD, it hurts to move it at all. Too often health care professionals dismiss all complaints of abnormal pain, feeling the patient complains too easily. Some patients do complain a lot, but RSD has specific physical findings that should alert the health care professional and the patient to the possibility of a more serious problem.

Thermography is one helpful test in diagnosing RSD in this early stage. It measures differences in skin temperature, hopefully pinpointing where the blood flow is being impeded. Nerve blocks are also used to diagnose early RSD. If the patient experiences relief with a sympathetic nerve block, that is a good indication RSD is present.

If RSD is caught at an early stage, the success rate is very high. Marcie, fifteen, hyperextended her shoulder while trying to catch a line drive, and the shoulder became red, hot, and swollen. She went to an orthopedic surgeon who took X rays and determined she didn't have any broken bones, but she did have a sprained shoulder. The shoulder continued to hurt and the pain began moving down her arm to the elbow, so she went to see her chiropractor, who suspected early RSD and sent her to a multidisciplinary pain center. There, the diagnosis of RSD was confirmed and an anesthesiologist administered two pain blocks. The chiropractor followed up with manipulation therapy, and the orthopedic surgeon monitored the sprain. Within three weeks, Marcie's symptoms completely disappeared, and she went back to playing softball but avoided line drives.

If RSD goes untreated, it enters the second stage, the dystrophic stage. *Dystrophic* means abnormal behavior, and that is exactly what continues to occur in the second stage. The major arteries still function, so the affected area gets enough blood to keep it alive, but the tiny artery branches, called arterioles, constrict so that the area around the injury is deprived of nutrients. Nerves, muscles, and bone in the area don't receive enough oxygen, vitamins, minerals, proteins, and other essential nourishment. Lack of nutrients causes nerve, muscle, and bone pain, which explains the symptoms. But the abnormal blood flow now isn't just restricted to the area of the injury; the vessels clamp down in the entire area. Instead of the wrist hurting, the entire forearm, or even the entire arm, may hurt.

This is where diagnosis gets complicated for the health care professional. Doctors are trained to look for a specific nerve or group of nerves that is causing a problem, but RSD doesn't follow normal nerve patterns. An ankle injury could result in RSD creeping up the entire leg to the hip.

Bone scans, nerve blocks, sweat response tests, and skin conductance response tests can be used to help diagnose RSD in the second and third stages. Bone scans are X rays that identify RSD by exposing changes in the way a marker drug appears in the bone or joint. RSD patients produce too much sweat, and the sweat response test measures these differences. Areas of RSD can conduct electricity differently than the rest of the body and the skin conductance test measures that flow.

RSD can be treated in the dystrophic stage. A delay in treatment decreases the success rate, but this stage of RSD can be cured.

Bill, fifty-three, worked as a lineman for an electric company. Because he used the same movements often in his work, he developed carpal tunnel syndrome, a wrist injury, and he also had pain in his hand. An orthopedic hand surgeon corrected the carpal tunnel, but the surgery lasted longer than the usual twenty minutes because he also removed some inflamed tissue from the tendons.

Bill had the usual postoperative pain and went to physical therapy, but he did not improve. The hand remained swollen for four months and continued to hurt. The surgeon suspected Bill had RSD and referred him to a multidisciplinary pain center. His hand was swollen and cold, and touching it or moving it was very painful, confirming a diagnosis of RSD in the second stage.

An anesthesiologist performed a series of thirteen stellate ganglion blocks over a course of two months. The stellate ganglia are a group of nerves in the neck that control the sympathetic nervous system on the face, arm, shoulder, and upper chest on either side of the body. These blocks were accompanied by physical therapy and medications, including calcium channel blockers, antidepressants, and NSAIDs. After the two months, Bill was at least 80 percent better and was able to return to work and stop taking his medications.

In the third, or atrophic, stage, the lack of blood supply begins to cause permanent damage to the muscle, nerves, and bones. The muscle begins wasting away and the bone becomes more brittle and is more likely to break. In some patients, the RSD at this stage affects the entire limb and they lose use of it. In some rare cases, the patient loses sensation in the limb, which helps relieve the pain, although the damage continues.

The atrophic stage is slow to develop and may not show up for years following the injury. RSD is much more difficult to treat at this stage. Sometimes the pain practitioner can only treat the pain, and may not be able to return full function to the limb.

JoAnn, fifty-one, broke her shin bone in a motorcycle accident. The bone was set surgically, but she developed osteomyelitis, an infection in the bone, which was successfully treated with antibiotics. But the pain didn't stop when the infection and the bone healed, and she began showing symptoms of RSD with increased sensitivity, a cold leg, reduced range of motion, and pain that traveled up her leg. Eventually, the RSD spread until she had pain even above the knee and down to her ankle.

JoAnn tried physical therapy for six years, chiropractic care for ten years, a TENS unit (transcutaneous electrical nerve stimulator, which uses a nine-volt battery to deliver electricity to the painful area, interrupting the pain signal) for twelve years, biofeedback, nerve blocks, acupuncture, and multiple medications, none of which cured her pain. For ten years, she was on chronic narcotic therapy and antidepressants.

JoAnn was fitted with a brace because her muscles had started wasting away, and she had to use a cane to walk. Sixteen years after the initial injury, she was referred to a multidisciplinary pain management center by a doctor who specialized in addiction. JoAnn had tried to wean herself off the narcotics with the help of her addiction doctor, but the pain was too intense for her to quit taking the medicine. Other medications had been tried, but they didn't help the pain. By the time she was referred to a pain center, the narcotics were no longer as effective, and she was having more difficulty walking and functioning.

At the pain center, she was diagnosed with RSD and an anesthesiologist administered nerve blocks, but she didn't experience any long term relief. JoAnn began having low back pain, and there was concern the RSD was spreading.

Her anesthesiologist consulted with her primary care physician and psychologist, and all agreed she was a good candidate for a spinal cord stimulator (SCS). An SCS uses small electrodes in the epidural space next to the spinal cord to block the pain signal from reaching the brain. The temporary stimulator reduced her pain 80 to 90 percent and she was able to stop all of her pain medications, so a permanent one was installed. With the permanent SCS, JoAnn was able to discontinue all medication and walk without a brace or cane. The RSD had aggressively traveled up and down her leg, but was finally halted.

RSD AND THE MIND

Unfortunately, RSD causes more than just physical problems. The continual pain and the loss of the ability to function normally takes its toll on the mind as well. Some studies suggest that up to 75 percent of RSD patients in the second and third stages are depressed, while individual practitioners maintain that virtually all of their untreated RSD patients develop psychological problems, including anxiety, phobias, irritability, agitation, and depression. Psychiatric studies have shown that about 90 percent of RSD patients did not have psychological problems before they had the pain, but that the physical deterioration and pain damage the mind as well as the body.

For most pain sufferers, psychological techniques can help control pain. Studies show that about 33 percent of pain patients who are given a placebo show improvement. But in RSD patients, only 10 percent report any improvement with a placebo. With RSD, the pain is so overwhelming, so intense, that the mind can't help as much. These patients have nerve, muscle, and bone damage, which makes their pain more difficult to control psychologically *and* physically.

What You Can Do

RSD isn't as well known as some other types of chronic pain, so if you suspect you have it, make certain your health care practitioner is familiar with it. Don't be afraid to ask questions. If your practitioner isn't willing to take the time to answer your questions, it's time to find a new doctor. Because RSD is complicated and has so many side effects, it is often best treated in a multidisciplinary pain center.

RSD patients can help their chances tremendously by changing their lifestyle. Because RSD is caused by constricted blood vessels and starving tissue, anything that hurts circulation should be stopped. RSD patients must quit smoking. Smokers have a greatly reduced chance for successful treatment because smoking causes the blood vessels to clamp down even more. Avoiding cold temperatures also helps the RSD patient. Cold makes the blood vessels constrict even more, making the pain and the damage worse. Alcohol should be avoided, even though alcohol causes some blood vessels to dilate. When you drink, the blood vessels on the surface of the skin dilate, sending more blood to your skin, but the muscles actually get less blood, aggravating RSD. Alcohol also cripples the body's ability to regulate temperature, which can make the RSD site even colder. Alcohol reduces rapid eye movement (REM) sleep, the most restful and refreshing kind. When you're deprived of REM sleep, you're more tired and depressed the next day, two conditions the RSD patient has more than enough of, anyway. Caffeine appears to worsen RSD, also. There are no studies to show this, but caffeine is a stimulant that causes the release of chemicals that squeeze the blood vessels. Except for certain types of headaches, almost everyone with pain should avoid caffeine.

Capsaicin cream, which is available over the counter, might be used to decrease sensitivity on the skin and can help with deeper pain. Some RSD patients can't try it, however, because RSD has made their skin too sensitive, and capsaicin can be irritating. If the cream is too irritating (it is supposed to burn somewhat), place a paper towel soaked in milk over the area.

Another over-the-counter product that sometimes helps is the mineral magnesium, which is sold in the vitamin section of most pharmacies. It relaxes the muscles surrounding arteries, allowing more blood to reach the affected area. Melatonin, which is also sold in many pharmacies, appears to help some RSD patients sleep better.

A healthy diet is essential for anyone in the healing process. RSD deprives the injured site of nutrients so your diet should be as nutritious as possible. Fresh fruits and vegetables provide necessary vitamins and minerals, while low-fat dairy products, such as skim milk and cheese, help boost the body's calcium and magnesium levels. Milk products also contain tryptophan, an amino acid that helps in the healing process and allows more restful sleep. Science is learning more and more about the value of trace minerals, such as selenium and copper, and eating lots of whole grains and fresh produce provides the appropriate amount for the body. Trace minerals can be toxic in excessive doses, so it is best to get them from a healthy diet instead of from vitamin pills.

Other than changing your diet and habits, there isn't too much you can do to help RSD. This is a disease that needs professional treatment by someone who knows what they're doing. The wrong kind of treatment can actually make RSD worse and cause more permanent damage.

What Your Doctor Can Do

RSD is one type of chronic pain that requires aggressive, invasive therapy, and it doesn't generally respond to more conservative treatments. RSD alters the area it affects and causes physical deterioration. In many types of pain, once the cause of the pain has been treated, the area around it can return to normal. But in advanced stages of RSD, it is too late to undo the damage. This change in the body makes RSD difficult to treat conservatively.

Even in the first stage of RSD, aggressive therapy seems to work best. The tissue around the injury is deprived of nutrients and is being destroyed, and normal function must be restored so the area can heal. A multidisciplinary approach to the treatment of RSD is essential. Physical therapy may help some patients, nerve blocks may help some patients, but a combination of treatments has the highest success rate. RSD needs to be hit from all sides and it usually takes more than one method to beat it.

The first thing a doctor will do is decide what stage of RSD the patient has, which will determine where treatment begins. In advanced stages, more aggressive treatments will be tried sooner because more conservative treatments aren't as effective. One of the first things that will probably happen in the early stages is the patient will be placed on calcium channel blockers (CCBs). CCBs open up blood vessels, increasing the blood supply to the RSD area.

A new drug, gabapentin, which is actually an antiseizure medicine, has been shown to be effective in RSD. This drug works in the brain to help RSD, but researchers haven't discovered why. Another medication, baclofen, a muscle relaxant, helps with some RSD patients, probably by slowing down the sympathetic nervous system in the brain, but scientists aren't exactly sure how it works.

Many RSD patients don't sleep well, and when they do sleep, they don't have enough REM sleep, so they are sometimes placed on tricyclic antidepressants. This medicine allows a normal sleep cycle, and the patient wakes up refreshed and rested. It also works in the brain to reduce pain, but the exact mechanics are still unclear.

As with any medication, the patient needs to receive enough to discover if it works. A week to one month may be necessary to see if it will be effective. And all prescription medication must be taken according to the directions because the timing and dosage affects how well the medicine works.

Medicines are only the first step in treating RSD, and must be combined with physical therapy and nerve blocks. The goals of this second stage of treatment are to desensitize the area and improve mobility. Because the area is already extremely painful, sometimes nerve blocks must be administered to make therapy possible. Nerve blocks for RSD don't anesthetize the sensory nerves and block pain. Instead, sympathetic nerve blocks allow the body to bring in a fresh supply of blood, oxygen, and nutrients to the area. Sympathetic nerves regulate the blood supply, so by blocking them, they can't inhibit blood flow to the site. Remember, the pain from RSD comes from an area not getting enough blood, so if circulation improves, so will the pain.

In persistent RSD, an anesthesiologist may have to administer three, four, or five blocks a week to retrain the sympathetic nerves. And the course of treatment may take several weeks or months because, like training anyone or anything, it takes a while to get the message across.

The type of block will depend on the area that has RSD. Some anesthesiologists will use a tourniquet on the arm or leg and inject intravenous medicines, opening up blood vessels. Others use blocks, such as stellate ganglion blocks, thoracic or lumbar epidurals, or thoracic or lumbar sympathetic blocks, to achieve the same goals.

The stellate ganglia are a group of nerves in the neck that control the sympathetic nervous system for the head, neck, and arms. Anesthesiologists inject a local anesthetic and sometimes a small amount of steroid into the area to calm the sympathetic nerves. The steroids help reduce inflammation and might help the anesthetic effect last longer. The blocks can be painful and sometimes the patient receives a sedative beforehand.

Joan, twenty-nine, had carpal tunnel surgery (to relieve pressure on nerves in her wrist) on both wrists, and had no problem with the surgery on the right side. After the second surgery for her left side, though, she began having pain as soon as the splint was removed. Her entire arm, from armpit to fingers, had sharp, shooting pain with a numb, tingly feeling, and anything touching it hurt. Her surgeon prescribed physical therapy, but the arm was too painful to finish the sessions.

The pain became worse, and Joan switched from being left-handed to right-handed because she wasn't able to use her left hand as much. Her left arm became smaller as the muscles wasted away from not being used enough, and it was colder to the touch than her right arm. The fingernails on her left arm became brittle, and her arm hair fell off in patches. Her doctor prescribed NSAIDs, but they didn't help much, and after two years, her surgeon referred her to a multidisciplinary pain center.

An anesthesiologist gave Joan a stellate ganglion block as a test to see if it helped with the pain. It did, but the doctor told her there had been so much damage from the RSD that he wasn't sure further blocks would be much help. He placed her on gabapentin, an antiseizure drug that sometimes helps with RSD, and gave her another block. Two weeks later, she felt 30 percent better, so she was given one more, which gave her 75 percent relief. After another two weeks, the anesthesiologist administered one more stellate ganglion block, and Joan's pain disappeared.

Thoracic or lumbar epidurals place local anesthetic and perhaps some steroids into the space between the spinal cord and the ligaments in the spine. Every nerve except the sensory and motor nerves for the face passes through the epidural space before it goes out into the body. *Thoracic* refers to the middle twelve vertebrae in the back that protect the nervous system for the rib cage area. *Lumbar* refers to the bottom five vertebrae that house the part of the nervous system supplying the body from the waist down. Sometimes anesthesiologists use these epidurals to anesthetize the sympathetic nervous system, which carries the pain signal back to the brain. The anesthesiologist uses local anesthetic to numb the skin before inserting the needle. The procedure is mildly uncomfortable but should not be painful. Thoracic or lumbar sympathetic blocks are done under X ray because they are very selective and pinpoint exact nerves. These sympathetic blocks insert local anesthetic into specific sympathetic nerve groups, so they will relax, allowing more blood and nutrients to flow to the RSD area. This procedure is more painful than epidurals because the injections have to go deeper and pass through muscle. The skin is numbed before the shot and the patient is frequently given a sedative to ease discomfort.

Because of the nature of RSD, surgery won't work. Patients have asked doctors to cut their hands, arms, or legs off to stop the pain, but all it will do is send the RSD farther up the limb, giving the stump the same symptoms the arm, hand, or leg once had.

Cutting the nerves might seem to be an option, but even when surgeons cut the sympathetic nerves, the relief is generally only temporary. The nerves reroute and cause the same problems they did before. Years ago, surgical removal of the sympathetic nerves was about the only option. Today, doctors are trying radiofrequency to kill sympathetic nerves, but no long term studies have been done to determine if this technique works any better than surgical removal of the nerves. Radiofrequency has the advantage of being done on an outpatient basis and is safer than surgery and is discussed more fully in chapter 13.

As with the medicines, you have to be patient as treatment begins. RSD didn't happen overnight, and it probably won't go away overnight. Nerves have to be retrained and the damaged tissue repaired as much as possible. The amount of time since the initial injury, the types of treatment tried, and the severity of the disease all affect how long it takes to show results. It could take days for someone in the first stage or months for someone with more severe RSD.

If after repeated therapy with medicine, physical therapy, psychological help, and blocks, the pain still persists, then it is time to think about more advanced technology, such as spinal cord stimulators (SCS) or implantable pumps. These options are discussed more fully in chapter 13. Narcotics may also be an option at this point, if other methods simply don't produce the desired results, but they are a last course of treatment, not one of the first.

Patients with RSD are doubly cursed because the disease is so difficult to diagnose, and it is also one of the most painful syndromes. There are no definitive tests to diagnose it and no universal symptoms to alert the doctor that he is dealing with it. But new technology and treatments give hope where once there was none. By combining knowledge and methods, health care practitioners and patients now have a fighting chance.

CHAPTER 5
ARTHRITIS

I don't deserve this award, but I have arthritis and I don't deserve that either.

Jack Benny

NOBODY DESERVES ARTHRITIS, but almost everyone gets it. Some just get a few aches and pains as they age, while others are crippled by it. There are more than 100 types of arthritis, some nastier than others, but all inflame and sometimes disfigure the joints. Even though everyone gets arthritis at some point, it is a mysterious process because it serves no useful purpose, perpetuating itself when common sense says the inflammation should have stopped. If you bruise a muscle, the injury heals and the inflammation stops. But in arthritis, it just keeps going. Actually, it is very nonuseful because it cripples the body and slows it down, draining energy from healthy parts.

The term *arthritis* means joint inflammations, but that doesn't identify the specific kind, although it usually means osteoarthritis. Osteoarthritis, or degenerative joint disease (DJD) is the most common form of bone pain. As we age, everyone develops arthritis as the joints wear out. Ninety percent of us develop some kind of arthritis by the time we're forty. Although we don't always feel any pain yet, the disease started with microscopic lesions in the cartilage by the time we reached twenty.

Cartilage pads the end of the bones, protecting them from rubbing against each other, but this cartilage is not as strong or as durable as the bones it protects. It's like the tires on a car, the asphalt and the pressure of the moving vehicle are stronger than the tire, so it eventually has to be replaced. Unfortunately, you can't go down to your neighborhood store for a new set of cartilage, so arthritis develops.

Arthritis begins at the edge of the cartilage where it meets the bone and periostium, the protective covering of the bone, causing inflammation as the cartilage begins flaking around the edges. As the disease progresses, the bone fights back by growing around the cartilage. Cartilage has lots of nerves just under the surface, and when the joint moves, this new bone rubs those nerves, causing pain. That's why it is so important that you continue to use the joint. If you stop using it, the bone invades even more of the space where cartilage used to be, increasing the pain when you do use it.

Another type of arthritis, called secondary arthritis, is caused by trauma, when an injury breaks down the cartilage instead of time and pressure. Although osteoarthritis is a slow process, arthritis caused by trauma can happen quickly, the injury damaging an otherwise healthy joint. Symptoms and treatment are the same for secondary arthritis, but as the cartilage repairs itself, scar tissue forms, which isn't as strong or as smooth as the original, so that even though the joint heals, it is never as good as it was before the injury, just as in osteoarthritis, where the joint is never the same again.

One common complication of arthritis is chondromalacia, a fancy term for softening cartilage that is usually seen in younger people, particularly in the knee joint. In chondromalacia, the cartilage flakes not only on the edges, but throughout the entire joint surface, exposing the bone beneath. Overweight patients are more likely to develop this complication because the extra weight puts more stress on the joint. But some patients who aren't overweight develop it, having the bad luck of a hereditary predisposition to the disease. Athletes, particularly professionals or overzealous amateurs, can also develop chondromalacia because they repeatedly put a lot of strain on the same joint over and over.

What You Can Do

Pharmacies sell literally thousands of over-the-counter (OTC) devices and medications to help with arthritis, from liniments to aspirin to back braces. With mild osteoarthritis, almost anything that helps is just fine. If an OTC nonsteroidal anti-inflammatory (NSAID, which reduces inflammation) coupled with a heating pad gives relief, then that's what you should do. Never combine medications, though, without reading the ingredients first and checking with a pharmacist or your doctor. Some patients will accidentally overmedicate themselves by taking two different brands of the same medicine, when such a high dosage could be toxic. Also, always check with your doctor or pharmacist before mixing OTC medicines with prescriptions to avoid any harmful interactions.

Some patients report relief when taking glucosamine, an aminosugar that helps build tissue, which can be bought in many health food and drug stores. It is sometimes combined with chondroitin sulfate, a nutritional supplement also available from health food and drug stores. It can take weeks or months for this method to work, so don't give up after a few days.

Capsaicin cream seems to help many arthritis patients, the power of the chili pepper easing aching joints. Always wash your hands after applying it, and if the burning on the skin becomes too much, soak a paper towel with milk and place it over the site. Capsaicin has to be used regularly for the best effect and can take up to a month to be effective, so don't give up after one or two applications.

Exercise is vital for the osteoarthritis patient to keep the joints moving and prevent further damage. Like with OTC medicines and devices, you can experiment and see what works best for you. If twenty minutes on a stationary bike helps knee pain, for example, then you should keep doing that. Swimming is one exercise that is good for almost any osteoarthritis patient, keeping weight off the joints while the muscles get a workout. Just walking in the pool, as well as water aerobics, give the same benefit.

High-impact exercise isn't going to help, however, because the pounding will only worsen the disease. A marathon runner, for example, with osteoarthritis in her knees should switch to some other form of exercise, such as cycling, that isn't going to stress the joints so much.

The Arthritis Foundation suggests patients exercise every day, and if the pain from exercising lasts longer than two hours after you're done, go see your doctor. Cutting back on exercise is okay if it is too painful, and you might want to see your doctor to have an exercise program designed for your needs. Balance exercise with resting, and be careful not to overdo it and cause more damage to the joint.

Applying heat or ice packs to the sore joint often reduces swelling and helps with the pain. Be careful, though, not to get the skin uncomfortably hot or cold. Cold packs can damage the skin if left on for too long, and because cold numbs the skin, you may not feel it causing frostbite.

Obese patients have the toughest time with osteoarthritis because they put extra weight on painful joints. Try carrying a twenty-five-pound sack of dog food around the house, and you'll get an idea of why maintaining a healthy weight is so important for the arthritis patient.

As with all forms of pain, smoking and alcohol only make it worse. By constricting blood flow, they prevent healing and increase pain. Caffeine, too, increases pain by constricting blood vessels.

Support groups often help the osteoarthritis patient, but it's very important to get the right one. One negative person can bring down the atmosphere of the entire group. Be especially cautious of groups run by lay people. Counselors and other mental health care professionals often run the best groups. The right support group offers tips on how to deal with the pain, and sharing suggestions and stories will probably help your mental health.

What Your Doctor Can Do

One of the first things your doctor will do is to make sure the pain is osteoarthritis and not something else. He will probably order an X ray, and if there is any fluid on the joint, he might use a needle to draw off some of that fluid and send it to the laboratory for analysis, which will help pinpoint the exact cause of the pain. Analyzing the fluid will help the doctor determine what kind of arthritis you have, and an X ray shows any damage to the joint.

Because exercise is so important for the osteoarthritis patient, he will probably teach you exercises you can do at home or send you for physical therapy. A physical therapist can create an individualized exercise program that works for your pain and your lifestyle.

If over-the-counter medicines aren't doing the job, the doctor might prescribe prescription NSAIDs to reduce the inflammation in the joint. Tramadol (Ultram), a nonnarcotic painkiller, also often works well for arthritis pain. Sometimes, if the pain is persistent and nothing else seems to work, narcotics might be prescribed for short-term relief of pain. Tricyclic antidepressants are sometimes prescribed for osteoarthritis patients who have a hard time sleeping because of the pain.

Injecting the joint with steroids and a local anesthetic is sometimes done for flare-ups of pain. Steroids can almost always stop the inflammation, but they soften the cartilage and ligaments, so shots are usually limited to no more than three times a year. Although injections are a short-term solution, they might delay the need for surgery or narcotics, benefiting some patients.

Osteoarthritis is the number-one reason for knee, hip, and shoulder joint replacements. When nothing else works, a new joint may be the only choice, but an artificial joint never lasts as long or works as well as the original, so it's not a good idea to do joint replacement surgery in a young, active patient. The more use an artificial joint gets, the

quicker it wears out. Obese patients are also not good candidates for joint replacement because the extra weight
stresses the new joint too much. Often, surgeons require
overweight patients to lose some weight before making the
commitment to a new joint.

Surgery must be followed up with physical therapy to
teach the patient how to use the new joint and to make sure
they don't hurt it by doing the wrong kind of exercise.
Muscle tone around the joint may have deteriorated, and
must be rebuilt to support it.

RHEUMATOID ARTHRITIS

Rheumatoid arthritis inflames joints, too, but for different
reasons. This type of arthritis, which afflicts between two
and five million Americans, causes the body to attack its
own cartilage, mistaking it for a foreign invader, as if it
were the flu or the measles. Classified as an autoimmune
disease, rheumatoid arthritis sends the body's immune system to attack the cartilage padding the bones in the joints,
eating it away until the bones end up grinding against each
other.

Infection, whether from a bacteria or a virus, alerts the
body's immune system to send white blood cells so they
can surround the foreign body and destroy it. In rheumatoid
arthritis, the white blood cells surround the cartilage, trying
to consume it, mistaking it for something harming the body.

No one knows why the immune system goes awry in the
rheumatoid arthritis patient or what triggers the white blood
cells to launch a full-scale attack against their own cartilage, which they should be defending. Heredity seems to
play some part, but environmental causes, such as chemicals in the air, water, and soil, may also be responsible.
Some theorize that a bacterial or viral infection might con-
fuse the immune system, causing it to assault the body it
is supposed to protect.

The immune system in the rheumatoid patient does try

to defend the cartilage, even while it consumes it, as the body tries to deal with conflicting signals. Because the white blood cells eat the cartilage, the body makes more cartilage in defense, creating the large nodules that rheumatoid patients have around their joints. This new cartilage isn't as smooth and hard as the original, because it's being attacked as it's formed, resulting in the disfiguring bumps.

This type of arthritis also has different symptoms than osteoarthritis, and treatments vary. While osteoarthritis patients have stiff joints in the morning, the pain usually lessens with movement through the day. In rheumatoid arthritis, though, movement only makes the pain worse because it alerts the immune system, causing it to launch a fresh assault. This leaves the patient in a Catch-22 situation, where movement makes the pain worse, but not moving at all allows the joint to fuse, the joint sometimes disappearing completely on X rays.

Osteoarthritis sufferers might have pain in one joint, such as the knee, or in just a few joints, like the knee, elbow, and fingers, but the rheumatoid patient is not as lucky. Rheumatoid arthritis is relentless, progressing through the body, sometimes even attacking the organs, such as the kidneys or lungs. It is symmetrical, assaulting both hands, for example, instead of only one.

Women rheumatoid patients outnumber men three to one, and it usually begins when they are in their twenties to forties. Children get it, too, but only very rarely. Rheumatoid begins with the same symptoms as osteo, the patients reporting deep, aching pain that is sometimes sharp, but can be diagnosed through blood tests that pick up an antibody that occurs in most rheumatoid patients. Rheumatoid sometimes begins with symptoms of fatigue, weight loss, and low-grade fever.

What You Can Do

Choosing a doctor that specializes in rheumatoid arthritis is essential, because there are a lot of treatments available and you want someone who is familiar with all of them and understands their complications. Some of the treatments have serious side effects, and a doctor with specialized training will know what is the safest, most effective treatment. Ten to 15 percent of patients go into remission after treatment, while another 10 to 15 percent don't respond to any of the many treatments available.

Capsaicin cream, which is sold over-the-counter, sometimes helps with this type of arthritis. The cream needs to be applied regularly to be most effective, so don't quit if it doesn't help after one or two applications. Capsaicin is derived from chili peppers, so always wash your hands after applying it. It burns slightly when applied, but if the burning is too intense, soak a paper towel in milk and place it on the skin.

Support groups help some patients deal with this disease, but be careful to choose one with a helpful, supportive atmosphere. These groups, and your doctor, might also recommend self-help books that they've found useful.

Even though exercise doesn't make the joints feel any better in some rheumatoid patients, it does keep muscles from losing strength and tone. When muscles begin to atrophy, it can cause more pain, so the goal of exercise is to maintain mobility, keeping the muscles around the joint as strong as possible.

But sometimes, the patient prefers the joint to fuse, because once the two bone ends grow together and the cartilage disappears, the pain can be greatly reduced or eliminated. The patient can no longer move that joint, though, so while it might be desirable to have a wrist fuse, it isn't practical for joints you use more often, such as an elbow or knee.

Smoking and alcohol only make a bad pain worse for the rheumatoid arthritis patient by constricting blood vessels and slowing healing. A diet rich in whole grains and fresh fruits and vegetables gives the body essential tools to fight the disease. Taking calcium and magnesium supplements helps replace minerals essential to bone growth.

What Your Doctor Can Do

Medicines are the mainstay treatment in rheumatoid arthritis, with salicylates, the aspirin family, one of the first drugs usually tried. They reduce the inflammation and pain and are inexpensive, but they can cause stomach distress. Prescription NSAIDs reduce the irritation in the joint, decreasing pain, and are easier on the stomach than salicylates. The newer ones last longer, so they sometimes only have to be taken once or twice a day. Acetaminophen doesn't reduce inflammation very much, but it is a painkiller, and is sometimes prescribed with salicylates or NSAIDs. All of these take time to be effective and should be tried for at least one or two weeks before you decide if they are working for you.

Phenylbutazone is a prescription used for short term relief of rheumatoid flare-ups. It is a potent NSAID that helps calm the inflammation of an attack. You continue taking your other medications while this is working to calm the joint.

Deciding whether or not to take steroids is a big step for the rheumatoid arthritis patient. Steroids slow the immune response, hindering the white blood cells' attack on the cartilage, but they have lots of side effects, including water retention and an increased risk of cancer. Steroids aren't addictive, but once you begin taking them, you can't stop quickly because they prevent your body from making its own steroids. You have to slowly taper their use to give your body time to begin making its own and to let your immune system build itself up again.

Sulfasalazine, a sulfa drug that was originally used as an antibiotic, has fewer side effects than many arthritis drugs, but it doesn't work for as many patients as some of the other drugs. Scientists don't know exactly why it works for arthritis and why it works on some and not others.

Injecting gold salts has been used since the 1920s for arthritis but declined in popularity because of side effects, which include skin rashes and kidney problems. Doctors are beginning to use it again because an oral form has been developed that seems to be less toxic than the injections. You can't just eat gold to get the benefit, because your body won't absorb it, but when it is chemically bonded to a salt, it slows the autoimmune response, reducing its attack on the cartilage.

Another drug that restrains the immune system is penicillamine, which is not penicillin. This medicine works very well in some patients, but has serious side effects, including the development of autoimmune diseases, such as lupus. Penicillamine stops the immune response just in the joint, not in the entire body, but the patient and the doctor must decide if the risk is worth the benefit of the drug.

Hydroxychloroquine began its career as an antimalaria drug, but for reasons doctors don't understand, it can put rheumatoid arthritis in remission. Hydroxychloroquine isn't as toxic as some of the medicines for rheumatoid, but it's not effective for everyone. It can take up to six months for this drug to work, and the possible side effects include blindness.

Two other drugs that suppress the immune system are beginning to be used for rheumatoid arthritis, but one, cyclophosphamide, hasn't received approval from the Food and Drug Administration (FDA), and is still being evaluated. The other, azathioprine, is controversial because doctors haven't decided when patients should begin using it, whether earlier or later in the course of treatment. Studies show both drugs to be effective for this disease, but they can have serious side effects, including cancer.

Chemotherapy drugs, which were originally designed to fight cancer, are showing promise as a treatment for rheumatoid arthritis. Methotrexate is the one used most often to hamper the immune system so it doesn't destroy the cartilage in the joint. Patients receiving injections of this drug must be closely monitored with blood tests to pick up possible liver toxicity. Other possible side effects include kidney problems, nausea, diarrhea, and exhaustion.

All of the drugs listed above slow the progress of rheumatoid arthritis, reducing damage to the joint while easing the pain. Narcotics, however, do nothing to slow this disease, but can give relief from the pain. They don't preserve the joint and may actually lead to a decrease in the joint's function because they don't stop the disease. Narcotics are the only arthritis drugs that can be addictive; for more information on their benefits and side effects, see chapter 12.

Surgical removal of the nodules, or bumps, associated with rheumatoid arthritis isn't a long-term solution because they always grow back, but it can sometimes provide years of relief. Removing the nodules is often recommended for younger patients who aren't ready for a joint replacement. A forty-year-old, for example, may have nodules removed in her knee because an artificial joint will wear out while she's still young.

Sometimes, though, surgeons fuse the joint, eliminating a lot of pain but causing the patient to lose the use of the joint completely. When surgeons fuse joints, they don't remove them but hold them in place with pins or screws so they can't move, and eventually, the bones grow together. Fingers, wrists, and the spine are the most commonly fused joints.

Doctors prefer to keep the joint mobile if at all possible and will sometimes replace damaged joints with artificial ones that the body doesn't recognize as cartilage. Replacement surgery removes the old joint and substitutes a plastic one that does the job of the old without attracting the attention of white cells.

Replacement surgery is now commonly done for hands, hips, knees, feet, and shoulders, with elbows done less frequently. An orthopedic surgeon will usually replace the larger joints, such as the hips and knees, while surgeons trained in hand surgery usually replace finger and hand joints, and foot surgeons replace joints in the feet.

Surgery may not completely eliminate the pain in that joint, but it does lessen it, allowing the patient to get by with fewer medications. Physical therapy sessions after surgery retrain muscles that might not have been used much with the old, stiff joints and teaches the patient how to use the new ones.

ANKYLOSING SPONDYLITIS

While rheumatoid arthritis is primarily a women's disease, ankylosing spondylitis is almost always found in white men. This genetic disease causes inflammation in the tail-bone, pelvic bone, and lower spine, leading eventually to the joints fusing together.

On an X ray, ankylosing spondylitis looks like osteoarthritis, but a blood test can tell the difference. This joint disease progresses faster than osteoarthritis, usually fusing the joints in ten to twenty years, and there is nothing doctors can do to halt the progression. Once the joints fuse, the pain disappears, but it can leave the patient permanently bent over. Some mobility is lost once the joint fuses, but the patient can still function.

Because the joint inevitably fuses, treatment for this disease is limited to treating the symptoms. Physical therapy helps the joints fuse in the best possible position, as does maintaining an upright posture and sleeping on a flat surface, such as a board. NSAIDs are often prescribed for the pain, but occasionally narcotics have to be used.

Back surgery is almost never used for the ankylosing spondylitis patient, but sometimes the disease moves into the hips, and hip replacement surgery becomes necessary.

GOUT

Gout used to be called the disease of kings, because older, well-fed men seemed especially prone to this joint disease. Rich food and alcohol aggravate gout, increasing the amount of uric acid in the blood. Too much uric acid results in crystals forming in the joints, their sharp edges stabbing like little knives.

Drawings of elderly, plump men with their feet wrapped and propped on a cushion were the classic stereotype of this disease, but it also occurred in those who drank moonshine. Often moonshine was distilled in old car radiators, which contained lead that leached into the liquor, causing attacks of gout.

Today, doctors recommend you don't overindulge in food or eat large amounts of meat if you've had a gout attack. NSAIDs, whether in OTC or prescription strength, reduce the inflammation caused by the uric acid crystals, and sometimes doctors prescribe steroids for a few days until the attack passes. Steroids might also be injected in the gouty joint after the doctor has drawn off excess fluid buildup.

Sometimes doctors prescribe allopurinol, which causes you to urinate more uric acid, giving your kidneys more time to remove the extra. Allopurinol might also be prescribed to keep another attack from occurring.

PSEUDOGOUT

This joint disease is caused by crystals, too, but pseudogout is the result of calcium crystals instead of those from uric acid. This is often associated with osteoarthritis as the body tries to build up calcium in the injured joint, sending more calcium to the area than it can absorb, creating sharp-edged crystals.

Doctors usually discover pseudogout by using a needle to draw fluid off the inflamed joint and sending it to a laboratory for analysis. NSAIDs are used primarily to control the pain of an attack, and a short course of steroids may be prescribed to reduce the swelling more quickly. The drug colchicine reduces the concentration of calcium in the joint and shortens attacks. Colchicine can also be prescribed to prevent future attacks.

With more than 100 kinds of arthritis, it is impossible to list them all in this chapter. NSAIDs, physical therapy, and capsaicin cream are used for many types, but each individual kind of arthritis has its own specialized treatment, so it is important to see a specialist in joint disease.

Rheumatologists are internal medicine doctors who have specific training in arthritis of all kinds and can best direct a course of treatment. Sometimes a multidisciplinary approach to arthritis pain may be helpful if traditional methods are not offering adequate relief.

CHAPTER 6

SHINGLES AND POSTHERPETIC NEURALGIA

Stop it at the start, it's late for medicine to be prepared when disease has grown strong through long delays.

Ovid

SHINGLES AND ITS aftermath, postherpetic neuralgia, are the leading causes of suicide in chronic pain patients over the age of seventy. It is true nerve pain, with the virus traveling along the nerve, attacking it as it searches for a way to get out and spread.

Eighty percent of us get chicken pox as youngsters, suffering through a week of itching and fever, then recovering with no long-term effects. But the virus hasn't been killed by the immune system; it lies dormant in the nerves that run out of the spinal cord, waiting to ambush when the immune system weakens, turning into shingles. Striking about 300,000 Americans each year, it causes some people intense, short-term pain, while others never get rid of it.

Shingles occurs when the virus decides to attack again, killing cells where it was resting, and traveling along a nerve, like water through a garden hose, until it reaches the surface of the skin, where it forms small blisters. The blisters contain the virus, and when they pop, it is released into the air, reproducing itself after fifty, sixty, or seventy years of waiting. People with active blisters are contagious; they can give chicken pox to anyone who hasn't had it, so it is important to stay away from young children who might not have been exposed yet to chicken pox.

But the reverse is not true. Many people think that being exposed to chicken pox triggers a shingles attack, but it is a weakened immune system that sets off the disease, not exposure to the virus. The body already contains the virus and usually can't catch it a second time.

Shingles is an opportunistic disease, waiting for a chance to surface again when the body lets down its defenses. Those over fifty, and especially those over seventy, have an increased chance of getting the disease as the immune system ages. The body doesn't make as many white blood cells as it did when it was twenty years old, and the cells it does make aren't as strong as previous cells, leaving more chances for the shingles virus to erupt. White blood cells recognize foreign bodies, activating the immune system to defeat bacteria and viruses before they can take over. Cancer patients who have undergone chemotherapy or radiation treatment, which suppresses the immune system, have anywhere from a 2 to 50 percent chance of getting shingles. But the reverse is not true; getting shingles does not mean you are getting cancer. And organ transplant patients who are placed on steroids to keep the body from rejecting the new organ can also get shingles.

As the virus begins its search for the surface, chewing up the nerve path it is following, an intense, sharp, shooting, traveling pain begins. Patients with shingles almost always see a doctor right away because the pain is so bad, but in the first few days, shingles can be tough to diagnose if the blisters haven't appeared yet. It can take anywhere from two days to a week for the virus to make its way to the skin where the blisters show up, and in the meantime, the doctor might be confused about the cause of the pain and will try treating the patient for something else. But once the blisters appear, the diagnosis is tough to miss.

Half of all patients experience shingles on their chest, while 18 percent get it in the face, 14 percent in the neck, 14 percent in the buttocks and legs, three percent in the rectum and genitals, and one percent develop shingles all over their body. The blisters usually follow the nerve path, but sometimes there's only one or two, just as some children are covered with chicken pox from head to toe, while others get only a few blisters. Even before the blisters appear, though, the skin along the nerve path will be sensitive to the touch, sometimes to the point where it hurts too much just to wear clothes. Those over seventy tend to have greater pain than younger patients.

For some patients, the pain lasts up to a month, then the shingles retreat, sometimes leaving scars where the blisters erupted. Shingles can strike more than once, so weathering one attack is no guarantee it will be the last.

Shingles changes names to postherpetic neuralgia when the pain lasts more than four weeks. Half of patients over the age of seventy develop postherpetic neuralgia, where the pain can last forever if it isn't treated. The exact cause of the continuing pain isn't known, but it could be caused by the damage done to the nerve as the virus fought its way to the skin, or it could originate in the spine, where the virus first broke out of its dormant state. Early, aggressive treatment is the best way to prevent shingles from lingering.

What You Can Do

There is nothing to do to prevent shingles, but once an attack occurs, it's important to see a doctor right away, although that's usually the first thing a patient does because the pain is so intense. Most people will get better in four weeks with or without treatment, but studies show that early, aggressive therapy lessens the chance of developing postherpetic neuralgia. If after four weeks you still have pain and your doctor is using only one kind of medicine or therapy, ask about other approaches. If you don't feel you're getting better or getting enough pain relief, ask to see a specialist in shingles, such as a neurologist or an anesthesiologist, because it's important to defeat the virus in its early stages.

Everyone over the age of fifty should be sent to a pain specialist after the first week of shingles, and you may have to insist on getting treatment. Studies don't show which shingles treatment works best, so some doctors do nothing. Health maintenance organizations (HMOs) often balk at treating shingles because they say it isn't cost effective, but the risk of developing postherpetic neuralgia from shingles justifies early, aggressive treatment for this disease.

Cold compresses sometimes help with the pain, but heat rarely makes it better.

One complication of shingles is infection in the open blisters, so it's important to keep the site as clean as possible. Use an antibacterial soap and water, and always wash your hands before and after touching the sores. Remember, the blisters spread chicken pox, so don't share towels or other linens with anyone.

The blisters often itch, and you can apply lotions containing calamine or diphenhydramine hydrochloride (Benadryl) with a clean cotton ball. Creams containing salicylates (aspirin compounds) sometimes help with the pain and itching, also. Talk to your doctor before applying any of the over-the-counter hydrocortisone creams, because some scientists think the medicine in these creams will suppress the immune system in the blister site, making the attack worse, and possibly increasing the risk of infection.

Capsaicin cream is often helpful along the path of pain, but never apply it to the blisters. It is made from chili peppers, and it burns, so you don't want it touching an already sensitive site. Wash your hands after applying the cream or use a rubber glove to apply it so you don't accidentally rub your eyes with it. It won't cause any permanent damage but will hurt a lot. Capsaicin cream burns initially and if the pain is too much, soak a paper towel in milk and apply it to the area.

Health food stores sell pills containing adenosine, which some people say helps with cold sores. The virus that causes cold sores and the one causing shingles are related, so some people have tried the pills for shingles, but it hasn't been shown that it works. Some patients report that cough syrups containing dextromethorphan help with the pain, but there are no scientific studies to prove it. It could be that the dextromethorphan calms the nerve cells, keeping them from sending so many pain signals to the brain.

What Your Doctor Can Do

Two new antiviral drugs, acyclovir and famciclovir, generally shorten the course of shingles and decrease the chances of developing postherpetic neuralgia, with the most recent studies favoring famciclovir. An antiviral drug attacks viruses, like antibiotics attack bacterial infections. These drugs kill the virus and decrease the inflammation caused by shingles. They are very expensive, though, costing up to $200 for five to ten days of treatment. Either one should be given as soon as shingles is diagnosed to have the greatest benefit. Don't let your doctor do nothing, though, and insist you be given the best chance to avoid postherpetic neuralgia.

Drug companies work constantly on developing new antiviral drugs, so your doctor might have a different one he wants to try. Cancer patients or others whose immune systems have been weakened by disease might be given antiviral drugs that are not in pill form, but might be given intravenously (in the vein) and are designed to give these patients the greatest benefit.

Most shingles patients need short-term narcotics because the pain is so intense. For years, doctors thought narcotics didn't help nerve pain and prescribing them would only result in addiction, but now scientists know better. Nerve pain is the toughest to treat, and it doesn't respond to most pain medications, so narcotics are usually prescribed. But even narcotics don't work all of the time, so they might be combined with other medications.

Don't worry about addiction with narcotics for this type of pain because when you are in pain, the narcotics simply give relief, they don't give you a high. In a recent study of 10,000 burn patients, none became addicted to narcotics when they were administered for acute pain. In another study, four patients out of more than 11,000 became addicted when the narcotics were administered for acute pain. The benefit of pain relief far outweighs the tiny chance of addiction.

Any pain medication for shingles should work within twenty-four hours, so if you don't get relief quickly, tell your doctor so something else can be tried.

Tricyclic antidepressants decrease the chance of developing postherpetic neuralgia, although we don't know exactly why. There are a lot of side effects, though, and some people just can't take them. The side effects include sleepiness, disorientation, low blood pressure, dry mouth, and irregular heartbeat. The side effects seem to be worse in older patients.

Elizabeth, forty-three, was taking antidepressants after undergoing chemotherapy and radiation therapy for breast cancer. One day, she woke up with sharp, itchy pain in her left cheek and jaw, but with none of the blisters. When the rash developed, she went to the multidisciplinary pain center where she was being treated for pain following her cancer surgery. Her doctor diagnosed shingles and placed her on famciclovir for seven days. She was told to keep the rash clean, and that she was contagious. Within a week, the blisters cleared, and the pain got much better without her ever having to take narcotics. Early diagnosis, antiviral medication, and the fact she was already taking antidepressants when the shingles occurred helped keep her outbreak to a minimum.

Some doctors use steroids for shingles because they cut down on inflammation, although they don't decrease the chances of developing postherpetic neuralgia. Steroids probably reduce the risk of scarring from the blisters, and scarring might increase pain. Steroids should be combined with other medications, such as antivirals, antidepressants, and pain medications to have the best result.

Recent studies suggest that because the risk of postherpetic neuralgia is so high in those over fifty, and especially those over seventy, administering nerve blocks can be worthwhile because they reduce inflammation and can slow the attack on the nerve. Sometimes steroids are given with the local anesthetic in the nerve blocks, but either way, it seems to reduce the chance of postherpetic neuralgia. The blocks are given in the nerve path the virus has chosen, reducing pain as well as the course of the attack.

Acupuncture hasn't been shown to have any benefits in shortening attacks, but it does provide pain relief for some patients. Physical therapy gives some pain relief, also, but doesn't do anything to halt the attack.

Because the consequences of developing postherpetic neuralgia after a shingles attack are so devastating, shingles should be treated quickly and aggressively with a combination of treatments. Antivirals with antidepressants, pain medications, steroids, and nerve blocks have the best chance of stopping shingles before it becomes postherpetic neuralgia. Insist on prompt, aggressive treatment while it is still shingles.

Once postherpetic neuralgia develops, it is too late to try the antiviral medications because the virus has already done its damage. Giving antivirals four weeks after a shingles attack would be like giving antibiotics three months after a strep throat infection when the disease has run its course, leaving the damage behind.

As with shingles, treating postherpetic neuralgia with a combination of treatments gives the best results. Tricyclic antidepressants still give relief with this phase of the disease; antiseizure medications, like phenytoin and gabapentin, also help. Mexiletine hydrochloride, a medication for irregular heartbeat, acts like a local anesthetic from the inside, while nonnarcotic pain relievers, like prescription nonsteroidal anti-inflammatories (NSAIDs) and tramadol, give pain relief also.

If the patient has had the pain less than six months, a series of nerve blocks might be tried, the number depending on whether it helps or not. If the blocks temporarily halt the pain, and if the pain comes back a little less strongly, then the blocks are doing some good and should be continued. If the pain comes back the same or worse after the local anesthetic has worn off, then the blocks aren't doing enough good to continue.

Epidurals, which use local anesthetic and steroids, work for some patients. The patient is given a local anesthetic to numb the skin, and then the medicine is injected into the

epidural space, the area between the spinal cord and the
ligaments holding the spine in place. Epidurals fight postherpetic neuralgia at the root of the affected nerve, where it
comes off the spinal cord. More information on epidurals
can be found in chapter 13.

Ian, sixty-nine, woke at three A.M. one morning with
stabbing, traveling, aching pain in his left side, across the
rib cage. He didn't have any blisters, but experienced short,
intense bursts of pain that were aggravated by lying down
and by anything, even a shirt, touching the area. He went
to his primary care doctor, who saw the blisters, which had
erupted overnight, and prescribed acyclovir and acetaminophen with codeine for the pain.

Ian only took the pain medication at night so he could
sleep, and when the pain didn't get any better, his doctor
placed him on antidepressants, hoping it would shorten the
course of the disease. He couldn't tolerate the antidepressants, though, because they made him disoriented. The blisters disappeared, but after one month, the pain still wasn't
any better. His doctor sent Ian to a multidisciplinary pain
center where an anesthesiologist gave him an epidural
where the painful nerve originated in the spine, and the pain
disappeared and never returned.

Capsaicin cream might help even at this late stage, as
well as prescription local anesthetic creams that will numb
the painful area.

For postherpetic neuralgia that isn't helped by anything
else, long-term narcotics use might be necessary. Spinal
cord stimulators (SCS) are another last line of defense.
SCSs use electrical stimulation to block the pain signal and
are more fully described in chapter 13.

If everything else has failed, neurosurgeons might cut the
damaged nerves at their base in the spinal cord. This is a
very high-risk procedure, though, and the long-term success
hasn't been shown to be that effective, so it is usually reserved for those who are terminally ill from some other
disease, such as cancer.

Shingles and postherpetic neuralgia are devastating diseases, but early, aggressive treatment gives a good chance

of a cure, giving the damaged nerves a chance to heal. If your doctor doesn't seem to know how to treat it, immediately find someone else who does, because that's your best chance for beating this progressive, opportunistic disease.

CHAPTER 7
CANCER PAIN

Pain is a more terrible lord of mankind than even death itself.

Albert Schweitzer

C ANCER PATIENTS FEAR pain, especially dying in pain. Cancer and pain have been linked since man first named the disease, but as modern technology and methods change the way pain is treated, patients who demand pain control can live comfortably.

Between 75 and 90 percent of cancer pain can be controlled with a combination of conservative treatments and medications, with the remainder needing more high-tech methods, such as epidurals, nerve blocks, or intrathecal pumps, or perhaps cutting nerves or the spinal cord to block the pain. But the trick to cancer pain control is demanding it, because not all doctors are aware of modern medicines and treatments.

More than one million Americans are diagnosed with cancer each year, but studies show that at least 40 percent are not getting adequate pain control. In one study, 50 to 80 percent of cancer patients who were not in a hospice weren't getting the pain control they needed. Fifty percent of cancer patients in another study said that pain interfered with their quality of life and their ability to sleep.

Cancer is unique in the pain management field because there are so many potential sources for the pain, and the treatments themselves—surgery, chemotherapy, and radiation—can cause additional pain. Cancer patients often have more than one kind of pain; in one study, 81 percent reported pain in more than one area, with 34 percent saying they had three or more pain sites. Cancer pain can be nerve, muscle, or bone pain, or a combination, which is why it is often best attacked with a multidisciplinary approach.

Doctors and nurses are often taught to treat the disease and not the accompanying pain, but they are becoming more aware of the necessity of treating cancer pain. Before modern treatments, patients were often just handed pain pills to deal with pain. Reasons given for the undertreatment of pain include lack of training for health care professionals, fear of narcotics, state and federal regulations that make it tough to prescribe narcotics for the cancer patient, and insurance companies and HMOs either refusing to pay for adequate pain treatment or delaying treatment.

Your body makes cancer cells every day, but the immune system usually spots them and quickly kills them. Tumors are abnormal growths, any new cell that doesn't exactly resemble the one that made it. The body makes millions of new cells every day. Each new cell is supposed to have the exact DNA coding of its parent cell, but that doesn't always happen. Sometimes the mutated cell simply can't survive and dies on its own; other times, the immune system surrounds and destroys it.

Sometimes, though, the cell closely resembles the parent cell and doesn't change enough to attract the attention of the immune system, so it is left to grow. Fat cells occasionally reproduce in lumps, forming fatty bumps called lipomas. The cells look just like other fat cells under the microscope, but something in their genetic coding makes them clump together in unnatural ways. These fat tumors don't pose any threat to the body because they simply keep making more of these nuisance fat cells.

Lipomas are examples of benign tumor cells, cells that shouldn't be growing where they are but are not consuming or replacing normal cells. Benign tumors cause trouble, though, when they grow in a bad place, squeezing normal organs and tissues. One of the most common kind of benign tumors grow in the brain and along the spinal cord, where they put pressure on the brain or the central nervous system.

Even though a benign brain tumor isn't destroying normal tissue, its growth puts tremendous pressure on the brain and skull because the skull can't expand to allow this new growth the way skin can stretch to accommodate a benign tumor.

Malignant cancer cells do cause trouble because they replace normal tissue and interfere with the body's daily functions. The body often recognizes these cells as abnormal and tries to kill them, causing some people to feel tired and run a low-grade fever as the body turns its attention to the mutant cells. The cancer cells, though, use the body's own immune system to travel to different areas. Lymph nodes manufacture the white blood cells used in the immune system and are scattered all over the body. When they send these white cells to attack the tumor, the cancer cells often hitch a ride with the cells sent to kill them, ending up in the lymph node system, where they can use the lymph system as a path to spread to other parts of the body.

Metastasizing occurs when the cancer cells leave the confines of the original tumor and spread to other parts of the body. Certain cancers have a tendency to show up in specific areas; prostate cancer, for example, tends to metastasize to the bones. Doctors grade tumors based on their size, location, and how far they've metastasized from the original site.

Tumors don't have pain fibers and are not painful on their own, but as they grow, they push on surrounding nerve fibers. There are tumors that grow on nerves, but they are almost always benign. Organs in the body, like the heart, the lungs, and the stomach, have no pain fibers either, and a tumor in them doesn't hurt until it stretches the protective sac surrounding the organ. Tumors in the colon, for example, have to stretch the peritoneum, the protective covering of the organs in the abdomen, before the patient feels pain. Tumors in the bone have to grow until they stretch the periosteum, the protective covering of the bones or until they increase pressure inside the bone. Cancers of the blood, such as leukemia, cause bone pain because too many cells are created within the marrow (the interior of the bone, where blood cells are grown), stretching the periosteum, which has lots of pain receptors.

Shrinking the tumor often relieves the pain, so although most people think of chemotherapy and radiation treatments as treatment for cancer, they are also treatment for pain because they shrink tumors, relieving pressure on stretched nerves. Surgery can also be a method of cancer pain control because removing all or part of a tumor can reduce pressure on pain nerves.

What You Can Do

Doctors and nurses are often trained in treating cancer, but little training is given to controlling the pain that can accompany it. Cancer pain can be managed, but you may need one doctor for the cancer and another for the pain. No one can help you unless you ask for it. Patients need to accurately report their pain and they need to let the doctor know they expect treatment. Each cancer is unique, and each patient is unique, so you need to tell the doctor exactly what and how you're feeling.

In this era of downsizing medicine, it's important to remember that you have a right to good pain control. You have a right to see a pain specialist, but you might have to demand to see one. Always ask for a board-certified specialist who knows about modern pain technology.

Medicare offers all the treatments and techniques discussed in this chapter, so all Medicare health maintenance organizations (HMOs) must offer them as well. Don't let a Medicare HMO tell you they aren't available, because they are. This may not necessarily be true with other HMOs, because even though technology and treatments are there for your pain, it doesn't mean they are offered by your HMO.

Studies show that cancer patients often don't report their pain, and when they do, they often don't tell how much it really hurts. Reasons for this inaccurate reporting include:

♦ They don't want to be seen as a whiner.
♦ They're concerned about the side effects of the pain medication.
♦ They're afraid increasing pain means the disease is progressing.
♦ They want to save the pain medication for when they really need it.
♦ They're afraid of shots.
♦ They feel nothing can or will be done about the pain.
♦ They're afraid of becoming addicted to pain medication.
♦ They worry that pain treatment will interfere with the cancer treatment.

It is vital to keep cancer pain treated. Not only does it improve the quality of life, but studies show that people in pain heal more slowly. If your body is focusing on the pain, it can't focus on getting better.

You also need to choose a doctor who can help with your pain. A primary care doctor, such as a general practitioner or an internist, may not have enough training in pain management to help you. One recent study showed only 46 percent of primary care doctors had enough training to manage cancer pain. Some oncologists (doctors who specialize in the treatment of cancer) are better at treating pain than others. You might need both a doctor who knows about pain and one who knows cancer treatments. Demand to see a specialist in cancer pain or to be sent to a multidisciplinary pain center if you aren't getting the pain control you need.

Besides demanding the pain treatment you need, you also must give your body plenty of nutritional food to help it combat cancer. Cancer uses lots of energy, which is why one of the first symptoms of cancer can be unexplained weight loss. The cancer cells don't die off like normal cells, and they need energy to stay alive and multiply, so they grab everything they can to grow. Often, the body can't keep up. Tumors steal nutrition from normal tissue, weakening the rest of the body. A two-pound tumor can consume as much as 30 percent of the nutrition you eat each day. Normal cells need extra nutrition so they can stay healthy to fight cancer. This means you need to eat foods that keep your body strong. This does not mean you can eat all the cookies and ice cream you want. They're not doing your body much good because they don't have the vitamins and minerals your body so desperately needs. Lots of calories does not mean lots of junk food.

Nutritional supplements, such as Ensure, were developed for cancer patients and the elderly who may not be getting all the nutrition they need in their diet. But use them as supplements, in addition to meals, not as substitutes for meals. Liquid diet foods designed for those trying to lose weight are also a good source of nutrition, but again, don't use them in place of meals, but as snacks or a drink to go with meals.

Make everything you eat or drink count. Don't drink water, drink juice or milk. Protein from meat, beans, and milk helps prevent the wasting of muscles; vitamins and minerals keep the body strong. Cancer and its treatments sometimes alter taste sensations, so eat what tastes good to you.

If you think you aren't getting enough nutrition in your food, ask your doctor about taking vitamin and mineral supplements. Compare the amount of vitamins and minerals in several brands, and don't always assume the name brand vitamin is better than the store brand. Certain kinds of chemotherapy deplete specific vitamins or minerals, so be sure to check with your doctor to see if you should be taking extra amounts of those.

Drinking alcohol generally does more harm than good in cancer patients. Alcohol is empty calories and doesn't give your body any nutrition. It interferes with normal sleep patterns, and cancer patients need lots of rest as their body heals. If you're taking narcotics, do not drink any alcohol without first discussing it with your doctor because alcohol can increase the risks of side effects and decrease the effectiveness of the pain medicine.

Cancer patients should always check with their doctors before exercising. Exercise, in general, is good for the body, but you must work with the limitations of the cancer and its treatments. Your body is not only healing from the cancer, but from the treatments, such as surgery, chemotherapy, and radiation, and it probably needs more rest than it normally would. A physical therapist can often teach you exercises, such as isometric exercises, that help you increase strength without overtaxing your body.

Over-the-counter medications and liniments, such as capsaicin cream, might provide some relief, but you must always check with your doctor before using any of them. Acetaminophen, aspirin, and nonsteroidal anti-inflammatories (NSAIDs), such as ibuprofen, often help with cancer pain and can be purchased without a prescription. One study showed that 36 percent of patients with cancer that had metastasized to the bone reported good pain relief with NSAIDs. Chemotherapy and prescription medications might interact with medicines you can pick up at the drugstore, so never take anything without first asking your doctor.

If you have trouble sleeping, try melatonin or the antihistamine diphenhydramine hydrochloride (Benadryl). Unlike prescription sleep aids, these medications can be taken on a regular basis to help with sleep. As with all medicines, though, check with your doctor to make sure they won't interact with any cancer treatments or drugs.

Massage, biofeedback, and relaxation techniques you can learn from books all might help with cancer pain, and if your doctor approves and they make you feel better, then use them. Never substitute these therapies for cancer treatment prescribed by your doctor, but use them to help you feel better while you follow doctor's instructions.

Support groups have been shown to be very beneficial for some people, and you can locate one in your area through the American Cancer Society, mental health professionals, or by calling a local hospice. Support groups tend to do the most good when you use them to share ideas with other cancer patients and to learn about new research. Remember that every tumor is different, and every person is different, so although you might learn of new techniques, your doctor may not necessarily prescribe those techniques for you.

What Your Doctor Can Do

The first thing most doctors will do is to get the pain under control as quickly as possible. Easing the pain immediately is essential because pain depresses the immune system and doesn't allow you to think clearly. Treating cancer demands your full attention because you will be making decisions on what therapies to use and when to use them and pain distracts you from those decisions.

When a patient begins having pain, immediate relief almost always means medications, such as prescription non-steroidal anti-inflammatories (NSAIDs) and narcotics. The goal is to relieve pain quickly, get the patient comfortable, and then experiment with other pain control medications and techniques to keep him comfortable.

Some patients might require hospital admission at first, especially if the doctor wants to try intravenous medicine. This delivers medication right into the bloodstream so it can begin working quickly. Once the pain is under control, the patient can be sent home with appropriate medication.

The next step is to determine what is hurting and how to best treat it. The doctor must discover what is causing the pain because treatment will vary, depending on whether it is bone, muscle, or nerve pain and where the pain originates. For example, if a patient has a bone tumor that's causing pain, the doctor might prescribe oral medication and begin radiation treatments to shrink the tumor, eventually relieving pressure on the nerves. Cancer treatments, such as chemotherapy, radiation, and surgery, are also pain treatments because they get rid of whatever is causing the pain, but they can also cause pain; chemotherapy and radiation account for up to 25 percent of all cancer pain.

Chemotherapy is chemical therapy that shrinks or kills tumors. It can damage healthy cells, too, including nerve cells. Pain from chemotherapy usually affects the arms and legs, causing burning and tingling, and nerve damage can be permanent. If chemotherapy begins causing pain, tell your doctor immediately. Patients sometimes think that they must have that particular type of chemotherapy or the cancer will spread, but there are lots of different kinds of chemotherapy and your treatment can be switched to one that doesn't cause you pain. The longer you take chemotherapy that causes pain, the more pain you'll have.

Radiation treatments target specific areas, using X rays to attack the cancer. Because strong X rays are used repeatedly in a small area, the skin can become sensitive to the touch. The X rays can damage healthy tissue and nerves around the tumor, causing burning, aching pain that is sometimes deep and sometimes shallow, although it can take up to twenty years for the damage to cause pain.

Surgery might be used to remove the tumor, but it can also be used to remove bone or tissue to give the tumor more room so it doesn't press on nerves and organs. Surgery can also serve strictly as a pain control technique, cutting nerves, including those in the brain and spinal cord, that carry pain signals back to the brain. Surgery generally has minimum side effects, including the usual risk of infection, but it can cause some nerve damage. Your surgeon can give you a complete list of possible side effects.

Once chemotherapy, radiation, and surgery begin to work, the medication may be adjusted. As the reason for the pain decreases, the pain will get better, and the patient may not need as much medicine. When the patient is in extreme pain, all the medication is needed just to keep him comfortable, but as the tumor shrinks and the pain retreats, the higher dosage may now cause side effects. A patient, for example, may need 100 milligrams of morphine a day for a tumor pressing on a leg bone. As radiation shrinks that tumor, the patient may begin feeling sleepy because he is now getting too much morphine. Tapering the dose will keep the patient comfortable but decrease the side effects. Radiation and chemotherapy can take weeks or months to have any effect, so the side effects might sneak up on the

patient. Be sure to discuss any changes in how you feel
with your doctor so he can adjust dosages.

The most common ways to get cancer pain medication
are orally, transdermally (through the skin), rectally (as a
suppository), by injections, intranasally (nose spray or
drops), and intravenously. The easiest way to get medication is orally, by swallowing a pill. Most pain medications
can be taken this way, including NSAIDs, narcotics, nonnarcotic painkillers, antidepressants (to help you sleep),
steroids (medications that help with inflammation to ease
pain), antianxiety drugs, and antiseizure medicines used for
pain control.

Sometimes the cancer or its treatments may make it difficult to take oral medications because the patient is nauseous or has trouble swallowing. In those cases, medicine
can be delivered other ways, letting the patient get the same
benefit as if he had swallowed a pill. Some medications
work better or have fewer side effects when they aren't
swallowed. The Food and Drug Administration (FDA) recently approved using a lollipop with fentanyl (a narcotic)
to give medicine to young children, but it can also be used
for adults if they are too nauseous to take pills.

Transdermal medications are placed on a patch, releasing
the medicine into the skin, where it is absorbed by the body.
They provide a steady dose of medicine, but take twenty-
four to seventy-two hours to get fully into the bloodstream.
Narcotics can be delivered this way, as can high blood pressure medicines, which sometimes help with pain. Scopol-
amine, which helps with nausea, can also be absorbed
through patches.

Suppositories, which are placed in the rectum, allow
medicines to be absorbed through the lining of the bowel,
where they can then pass into the bloodstream. Suppositories shouldn't be pushed too high in the rectum, just an
inch or two, so they can be absorbed, and always take off
the wrapper before inserting them. Antinausea medications
and narcotics are sometimes given this way.

Injections may be given subcutaneously (just below the
skin) or intramuscularly (deeper in the muscle). Intramus-

cular injections are a bit more risky than those placed just beneath the skin because they penetrate deeper into the body, increasing their chances of hitting nerves and injuring muscles. If the needle is put in the wrong place, the injection could do more harm than good, so injections have more possible side effects than the other ways of taking medicine. They are generally given for flare-ups of pain, to get the medicine working quickly, and are usually given in a doctor's office, a hospital, or by a home health care worker.

The fastest way to get medicine into the bloodstream is by injecting it into a vein. Narcotics are most commonly delivered this way, but most medications can be given in the vein. Intravenous medicine might be given with a single shot, or it could be through an IV line already in place for chemotherapy or other medication.

Intranasal medicine is a fancy term for nose drops or sprays that get medicine to the top of the nose where it is absorbed through the nasal membranes. Some people don't like to take pills and prefer to take their medication this way; others might be too nauseous from cancer treatments to swallow medicine. Stomach acid destroys some medications, and delivering them through the nose sidesteps the stomach. Butorphanol tartrate, a nonnarcotic pain reliever, is often given in the nose, as well as calcitonin, which helps strengthen weakened bones.

Whatever method works for you, it is important to take the medication exactly as the doctor prescribes. If you have any side effects or you don't feel the medicine is working, immediately tell your doctor. Some patients are too good—they'll take a medicine faithfully even if it hurts their stomach or has other side effects. There are other medicines and other ways of taking them, so you can remain as comfortable as possible.

If the medicine is working and if there are no uncomfortable side effects, it is important to keep to the regular doses prescribed by your doctor. Everyone has a therapeutic window of medication, a level where the drug is doing the most good with the least side effects, and individual windows vary greatly. Keeping on a schedule helps maintain that therapeutic window, allowing you the greatest chance of keeping pain at bay.

Even this therapeutic window may not be enough for breakthrough pain, the kind that erupts following exercise or some other exertion. This pain usually lasts a short time but can require an extra boost of medicine to manage a flare-up. Patients should be given a rescue dose of medicine to keep at home, something that will tame breakthrough pain until it subsides or the patient can get to a doctor. Don't leave your doctor's office until you are absolutely clear what to do about breakthrough pain.

Cancer patients sometimes won't report an increase in pain because they're afraid it means the cancer is getting worse, but remember that pain is a warning system. Changes and increases in pain should be examined because it may not have anything to do with the cancer, and even if it does, the problem should be taken care of.

Sue, sixty-one, had cancer of the larynx that metastasized to her spine. She was well controlled with her medicine, but then she began having sharp pain in her lower back. Afraid it was only bad news, she didn't report the pain at first, but then it became so severe she had to go to the emergency room. There, doctors discovered she had a urinary tract infection, and after a few days of antibiotics, the pain disappeared. She was given extra pain medication until the medicine cured the infection.

One of the first pain medications your doctor might try are prescription NSAIDs and aspirin. Cancer can cause inflammation, and both these drugs help reduce swelling as well as relieve pain, especially bone pain in cancer patients. There are many different kinds of NSAIDs, and your doctor may have to experiment to find the one right for you.

Steroids are very potent anti-inflammatory drugs that keep down the swelling caused by tumors and can slow down the growth of some cancers. They might be used, for example, if a bone tumor were pressing on nerves and causing pain. Steroids can also cause some patients to feel more cheerful, and sometimes increase the appetite, both side effects that can be beneficial for cancer patients. But steroids also suppress the immune system, which is under attack already from the cancer, and can lead to infections, especially shingles. More information on steroids is included in chapter 11.

Narcotics are the most prescribed drug for cancer pain and the ones that cause cancer patients to worry most. This family of drugs is especially good for muscle pain, pain caused from tissue damage, and the pain caused by pressure on internal organs. Narcotics have been used for thousands of years as a mainstay to control pain, and they can work very well for many cancer patients with minimum side effects. Some narcotics are stronger than others, and doctors usually try the milder ones first because, in general, the milder the narcotic, the milder the side effects.

Patients worry about becoming addicted to narcotics, but the risk for cancer patients is so small, it's hard to put a number to it, though it probably runs in the range of one in 10,000. An addict is someone who takes medicine for an effect other than the one the doctor intended, and cancer patients almost always take narcotics for pain, not for recreation. Cancer patients just want pain relief that will let them get on with their lives.

Even if narcotics give you euphoria or make you disoriented, it doesn't mean you are addicted. You are simply experiencing a side effect of the drug. Most patients don't like those feelings because it makes them feel like they can't make decisions and because their mind wanders. Getting high on medications is not limited to narcotics. One patient couldn't take acetaminophen (Tylenol) because it made her feel drunk, while another couldn't take ibuprofen (Advil) because it made him lethargic.

Another concern of cancer patients is that they will build up tolerances to narcotics and then the medicine won't work if the pain increases. For the first few weeks or months when you begin taking narcotics, you do build up tolerances to the drug, so that you have to keep increasing the dosage to get the same level of pain control. But then the tolerance levels off, and your need for the drug stabilizes unless the pain changes, so that if your pain increases, your doctor can give you higher doses to help with the new pain after he determines that you need more medication. You also build up tolerances to the side effects, and usually the first to disappear are the euphoria narcotics sometimes cause and drowsiness.

Narcotics come in many forms, some stronger and some weaker, so the type you are taking can be changed if you need more or less medicine. Every medication has a half-life, the amount of time it lasts in the body. With narcotics, morphine has a shorter half-life, and has to be taken every two or three hours, while methadone has the longest half-life of the pure narcotics family. Pharmaceutical companies work constantly to improve the half-life of medicines so patients don't have to take them as often. New forms of morphine release the medicine at a slower, steady rate, so pills only have to be taken every eight to twelve hours. These longer-lasting medications are better for the patient because they keep the therapeutic level more even than shorter-acting varieties. Studies have shown that patients prefer taking fewer pills and are more likely to remember to take their medication when they only have to take it once or twice a day instead of four times or more.

These long-lasting narcotics dissolve slowly in the stomach and intestines, releasing the medicine gradually. It is very important not to chew these pills because that will release the medicine too quickly into the bloodstream. In Europe, patients are sometimes told to chew their long-lasting narcotic pills to get an extra boost for breakthrough pain. Once the pill is chewed, though, it isn't absorbed evenly, so it is better to take whatever your doctor has prescribed for breakthrough pain instead of chewing your narcotics.

Even though you will almost certainly not be addicted to narcotics, your body will become physically dependent on them, so it very important to not stop taking them quickly, but to taper off slowly. If you're taking oral medicines and become nauseous from cancer treatments, don't stop taking your oral medication, but ask your doctor to give you narcotics in another form, such as rectally, transdermally, or by injection.

Sometimes narcotics make you so sleepy that it's tough to get anything done. Demetria, fifty-five, had abdominal pain from stomach cancer that was well controlled with narcotics, but the drug made her constantly sleepy, keeping her at home. She was afraid to even walk to the mailbox because she frequently stumbled. She tried cutting back on the narcotics, which gave her more energy but also increased her pain.

The doctor treating Demetria for cancer sent her to a multidisciplinary pain center, where various treatment options were discussed. She liked the pain control she was getting with the narcotics, so she chose to stay with that and add another medication. The doctor placed her on a low dose of an amphetamine called methylphenidate hydrochloride, more commonly known as Ritalin, which allowed her to stay awake during the day, run errands, and lead a more normal lifestyle.

Small doses of amphetamines often counteract the sleepiness sometimes caused by narcotics. They don't affect the painkilling ability of the narcotics, and because the doses used are so small, the amphetamines usually don't interfere with a normal lifestyle.

Many cancer patients have the opposite problem of not being able to sleep enough. Increasing narcotics at bedtime just so you can sleep more is not a good idea because even though you are sleeping, overmedicating with narcotics doesn't produce restful sleep cycles. So doctors sometimes prescribe sleep medications in addition to painkillers.

One of the first sleep medications ever prescribed were barbiturates, but they are rarely used now because there are newer, better, and safer drugs on the market. Patients become dependent on barbiturates very quickly and have to be tapered off slowly because stopping abruptly can cause severe side effects, including death.

Another class of sleeping aid is the hypnotics, which include diazepam, marketed under the name Valium. These have the added effect of being an antianxiety drug as well as helping with sleep, but they are frequently only used for short-term sleep problems. Other common hypnotics are Dalmane, Restoril, and Halcion.

Tricyclic antidepressants allow normal sleep cycles while also helping with pain, especially nerve pain. These medicines usually take a week or two to begin to work, so don't expect them to have an immediate effect. They can cause annoying side effects, including a dry mouth and a groggy feeling in the morning, but these symptoms often disappear after taking the drug for several days or weeks.

Antidepressants may be used on their own to help with nerve pain, but they are usually teamed with narcotics or other medications. While narcotics are very good with muscle pain and pain caused by pressure on internal organs, they often don't work as well on cancer pain caused by a tumor pressing on nerves or other nerve damage. In many cases, the narcotics have to be supplemented or replaced with something else. Antiseizure medications can also be used by themselves or in combination with narcotics to help with nerve pain. Scientists aren't exactly sure why these antiseizure medicines work, but they modify nerve signals in the brain and it could be that they also modify the pain signals. Antiseizure medicines are frequently used to combat the nerve damage sometimes caused by chemotherapy and radiation.

With all these medications, it may seem the cancer patient will spend all his time taking pills, but your doctor will use only the ones you need and will try to keep your prescriptions to a minimum. The goal is to keep the cancer patient comfortable with as few medications as possible.

WHEN THE PILLS AREN'T ENOUGH

As with all pain, psychological counseling might help you deal with the pain and the cancer. Psychologists and psychiatrists can teach relaxation techniques that will help you cope with breakthrough pain and pain that comes and goes.

Sometimes these techniques make it possible for you to reduce your medication, which then reduces any chances of side effects. They also let the cancer patient feel more in control of his situation.

If you aren't getting the pain control you need from medication, then it might be time to consider technological techniques and devices. These methods work on pain from the neck down, but are more complicated to insert and maintain than simply taking medicines.

Nerve blocks destroy very specific nerves causing pain in clearly defined areas. A tumor pressing on a rib, for example, may be irritating a certain nerve, which can then be killed to stop the pain. Injecting the nerves with chemicals kills them, but doctors also use radiofrequency to destroy the painful nerves. Cryoanalgesia is sometimes used to freeze and kill the nerves, although they tend to grow back, but with fewer problems. These techniques generally use a local anesthetic in the area of the nerve, and the patient is given a sedative for the procedure. Surgery can also deaden nerves, but it isn't used as much now because it usually requires general anesthesia.

Severe pain might require more aggressive treatments, such as placing an alcohol compound in the spinal canal to kill nerves. This procedure can potentially cause serious complications, including paralysis. Neurosurgeons can sometimes cut nerves in the spinal cord that are causing pain. If a tumor is pressing on the spinal cord, for example, a neurosurgeon might cut the pain nerves above the tumors to ease the pain. The surgeon would only cut those nerves causing pain, not the ones that control movement.

For more broad-based pain, doctors can use epidurals and intrathecal pumps to stop the pain at the spinal cord before it gets to the brain. Epidurals have the advantages of being able to easily change the medicines to the spine, and doctors can put the tip of the catheter wherever the patient needs pain relief. Patients can push a button to release more medicine if they have breakthrough pain, and the epidural is easily implanted in an outpatient procedure with the patient awake. Disadvantages to epidurals are that they have a higher infection rate than intrathecal pumps because they need to be filled with medication every one to seven days, while intrathecal pumps can go weeks or months between fillings. Patients find epidurals sometimes aren't as convenient because the pump is carried on the outside of the body. Some patients get around that problem by injecting their medication directly into the catheter with a syringe and not using a pump at all.

George, sixty-five, had surgery, chemotherapy, and radiation to combat lung cancer and for two years did well. Then he developed back pain that radiated to his chest. Tests didn't show any cancer, and the pain seemed to follow the path of his scar from lung surgery, so doctors thought the pain might be caused from the radiation treatments and gave him NSAIDs to take during the day and mild painkillers to help him sleep at night.

When the pain didn't get any better, George was referred to a multidisciplinary pain center, where once more he was examined for cancer, but none showed up on any tests. Doctors there performed a series of nerve blocks to reduce the inflammation at the site and to help with the pain. He was also given four steroid epidural treatments where the pain radiated from the spine and for four months, George did well with occasional blocks and trigger point injections in his muscles for spasms.

When the pain began worsening, an anesthesiologist deadened the nerve in his back and chest that seemed to be giving George the most problem, but the pain then spread above and below that nerve. More tests revealed the cancer had spread to three vertebrae, and George told his doctors he was worried about being able to attend his daughter's wedding the next month. He was given narcotics but didn't like the side effects of sleepiness, constipation, and nausea, so an anesthesiologist gave him a permanent epidural pump, which completely relieved all of George's pain. One week after the epidural was implanted, he was sleeping well, eating better, and taking short walks, including one down the aisle with his daughter.

Intrathecal pumps deliver medicine directly to the spinal cord using pumps that are sometimes implanted in the body and sometimes placed on the surface of the skin. Pumps are placed under the skin only when they will be used longer than three to six months. Chapter 13 contains more complete information on epidurals, pumps, radiofrequency, and cryoanalgesia.

Barbara, sixty-one, had breast cancer that metastasized to the spine, causing several compression fractures (where weakened vertebrae break with normal usage). Radiation to shrink the spinal tumors didn't seem to help, and she was brought into the emergency room one day because the pain from the compression fractures had gotten worse.

Doctors admitted her to the hospital and gave her intravenous narcotics, but she was still in pain. They increased the dosage until she was almost comatose, but she still screamed if someone tried to touch her.

An anesthesiologist from a multidisciplinary pain center came to the hospital and put in a temporary epidural with narcotics, which immediately eliminated her pain. After a few weeks with the epidural, the doctor tried weaning her from it, thinking the pain from the fracture would be less by then. The pain was still intense, though, so Barbara was given an intrathecal morphine pump. The pump kept her comfortable and she was able to resume her previous activities and to receive chemotherapy.

Spinal cord stimulators (SCS) are almost never used for cancer pain because they work best on pain that stays in one place and doesn't change. Cancer pain varies frequently and can travel around the body, so other methods usually work better.

Cancer patients fear pain more than anything else, but modern technologies, medicines, and treatments offer a variety of solutions to individual pain problems. Treating cancer pain often requires more than one health care professional, with various specialties attacking the tumor and the damage it causes, coordinating their efforts for the benefit of the patient. Cancer patients need to be aggressive when pursuing help for their pain, and let their doctors know when something isn't working, becoming a partner in the battle against cancer pain.

CHAPTER 8
HEADACHES AND FACE PAIN

For all the happiness mankind can gain
Is not in pleasure, but in rest from pain.

John Dryden

Everybody gets headaches, with at least 70 percent of Americans getting one each year, and approximately ten million adults having headaches for more than 100 days in any year. We lose $15.7 billion in productivity every year from headaches, with working mothers having the highest percentage of days lost to this common malady.

Humans get headaches because that's where the brain is, the command center for the entire body, sending and receiving signals on everything and anything you're doing or feeling. This command center must be protected, so it is surrounded by sensitive nerves, bone, blood vessels, and muscles.

The brain itself can't feel pain. Surgeons can operate on the brain with no anesthesia, as long as they avoid certain sensitive arteries and three of the twelve cranial nerves, which do feel pain. However, the membrane protecting the brain and the spinal cord, the dura mater, is loaded with nerve fibers that are very sensitive to stretching and pulling, warning the body when anything attempts to invade the brain.

The skull protects the brain, surrounding it and the dura mater with a sturdy bone shell designed to keep foreign invaders out and the brain in place. Bone doesn't give, though, and can't expand if something on the inside, such as an enlarged blood vessel or a tumor, presses against it. Bone protects the brain, but it could also injure it if the brain bumped against it, so a cushion of liquid, called cerebral spinal fluid (CSF) surrounds the brain, protecting it from sharp bumps against the bone. CSF acts like the white part of an egg, cushioning the yolk so it doesn't break against the shell when the egg is moved.

In addition to the nerves in the head protecting the brain, the face contains many sensory nerve fibers to warn of danger and protect against foreign invaders. Most of these are in the tongue and mouth to guard that gateway to the body, but the nose contains a lot, too, since the sense of smell warns of many dangers.

All this protection for the brain and body means there are a lot of ways for your head to hurt. Headaches can be caused by intracranial (inside the skull) pressure, where something is pressing against the bone barrier. Blood vessels filled with blood can press on sensitive nerves in the dura mater that can't move out of the way because of the confined space. Tumors can cause pressure inside the skull, as can infections in the several pools of blood located throughout the brain. Anything that disrupts the delicate balance of the brain and its surroundings can cause a headache.

The skull is surrounded by the periosteum, a protective membrane, and like the dura mater, it has plenty of nerve fibers to alert the body when something is too close to the bone. Tensed muscles can pull or stretch the periosteum, causing the head to hurt. Blood vessels can open up, pressing on nerves on the outside of the skull, while blood vessels that clamp down decrease blood flow to the muscles, causing pain.

Headaches can also be caused by the other organs sharing the head, such as the eyes, ears, nose, mouth, and jaw. Diseases, infections, or malformation of any of these can cause headaches.

Because the brain is the command center, relaying information and messages throughout the body, almost anything that affects the body can trigger headaches. Food allergies, diet, infections, diseases, chemicals in the environment, stress, light, and just about anything that affects your body or mind can irritate nerves in the head, causing headaches.

Add to that the fact that most times the exact cause of a headache can't be seen on medical tests or exams, and you can see why headaches are such a mystery for doctors and patients alike. Almost anything can cause a headache and finding the root of that cause is usually the key to treating it, so the doctor and the patient often have to become detectives, tracking down what triggers a headache. That's why taking a thorough patient history is such an important part of any headache treatment.

Martha, forty-four, began having sharp pains in her head that didn't respond to over-the-counter (OTC) medicines, such as aspirin or acetaminophen. After several weeks, she went to her doctor who asked questions about her headaches and when they occurred. She began keeping track and realized the headaches were always worse at home and became better when she was out. She had her house tested and found there was a small amount of carbon monoxide leaking into her home from a heater. Breathing the carbon monoxide decreased the amount of oxygen in Martha's blood, causing her blood vessels to swell, pressing on nerves in her head. The heater was repaired, and Martha's headaches disappeared.

TYPES OF HEADACHES

Muscle tension headaches are the most common type of headache, but most people who have them never see a doctor. The word *tension* here refers to tension in the muscles, causing them to constrict blood vessels, reducing blood flow to the head. Tensed muscles can also pull and tighten nerves, which signal their distress as a headache. Tension headaches range from merely annoying to extremely painful, and the pain may vary during the headache, which can last from several hours to many days.

These headaches are often caused by stress, which makes muscles tense in preparation for defense or attack. The body isn't well equipped to deal with the everyday stresses of a hectic job or crying babies or a long commute, and tenses muscles, readying them to react to the cause of the stress. But we rarely need to react physically to stress, so the muscles don't relax, and they wind tighter and tighter.

If you're watching an action movie or a thriller, your muscles don't realize that the stimulation poses no danger, that it is only a visual image, so they tense, prepared to respond as you see car chases and other mayhem on the screen. When the movie ends and the stress disappears, the muscles relax, often leaving you with an exhausted feeling. The same thing happens with everyday stress, except the muscles don't get a chance to relax because the stress continues. The next time you're in the middle of an exciting movie, try to remember how those tensed muscles felt, and you'll get an idea of what's happening to muscles causing some tension headaches.

Not all tension headaches, though, are caused by stress. Anything that injures muscles can cause a tension headache, and it doesn't have to just be the muscles surrounding the neck and head. Sometimes injured muscles as far away as the lower back cause a headache by disrupting other muscles, the effect rippling up the body like a trail of falling dominoes. Metabolic disorders, such as an imbalance in natural hormones, low blood sugar, dehydration, and eating or smelling noxious chemicals create tension headaches. Diet can also cause tension headaches, with changes in food disrupting the chemical balance of the muscles.

Because many people associate tension headaches with stress, patients often don't seek treatment, thinking there is nothing that can be done. However, there is plenty that can be done for tension headaches, even those brought on by stress. Tracking down the source of the headache is always the most important part of the process, and once that is located, treatment can begin.

Sometimes not much can be done to alleviate the source of stress. The chief executive officer of a company may not feel he can switch jobs even if his position is giving him headaches, so he'll have to learn other ways to deal with the stress. A mother with two or three young children can't just take a two-week Caribbean vacation to get away from midnight feedings and earaches, but she can learn how to redirect her stress to give her muscles a rest. Exercise, bio-feedback, physical therapy, diet, and massage are just a few of the things that can help tension headaches caused by stress. For injured muscles, physical therapy, chiropractic care, exercise, medications, and muscle injections might give relief. Treatments are more fully discussed later in this chapter.

Migraines are the second leading type of headaches, causing about 30 percent of headaches, with their legendary pain described in texts dating back to ancient Greek and Roman times. Migraines are vascular (referring to blood vessels) headaches, triggered by pressure changes in the blood vessels. Usually, these types of headaches begin with a decreased blood flow to the head, then the blood flow increases, pumping too much into the confined space of the brain.

Unlike tension headaches, migraines usually fall into a pattern and appear to be hereditary. People who suffer from migraines can often predict a headache before it appears, and they might know how long it will last and its intensity. These headaches are broken down into two types: those that usually cover only one-half of the head and are preceded by an aura, and those that don't have an aura and can cover both halves of the brain or just one side. Auras can be a change in vision, a strange smell, or simply an unfamiliar feeling, but they warn the patient that the headache is approaching.

About 75 percent of migraine sufferers are women. Some get headaches on a regular basis; others only get one or two a year. Approximately half of those with migraines vomit from the pain, and 85 percent get nauseous. Seventy percent have muscle tenderness on their heads, while about half suffer visual problems, especially sensitivity to light.

Migraines are still a mystery, even though they've been

known for thousands of years. They can last up to three days, although most last only a few hours, and they peak in intensity, then the pain slowly subsides. Scientists don't know what causes them, but it could be some kind of biological trigger in the body's cycles.

For years, patients didn't have much hope when it came to migraines, but today, new medications offer relief. Many people still think nothing can be done for these debilitating headaches, and it is estimated that up to half of migraine sufferers never even see a doctor.

Cluster headaches are the third most common type of headache, accounting for less than 1 percent. They were thought for years to be vascular in origin, like migraines, but some studies are showing they might originate outside the brain, perhaps as tension headaches, but no one really knows what triggers these excruciating headaches. Unlike many migraine and tension headache patients, cluster headache patients almost always see a doctor right away because the pain is so intense.

Cluster headaches tend to last fifteen minutes to three hours, stay on one side of the brain, and they can occur from one every few days up to eight a day. They don't give any warning like migraines, but they always have another symptom, such as a runny nose, watery eyes, sweating, or drooping facial muscles that accompanies the headache. These headaches tend to build quickly, then taper off. Nausea and visual problems are not as common with cluster headaches. About 85 percent of those with cluster headaches are men. Cluster headaches don't usually begin before the age of twenty, and they tend to lessen or disappear after the patient is in his sixties.

The only known trigger for cluster headaches is alcohol, but some studies suggest allergies, smoking, certain foods, or bright lights might also contribute to them. Nitroglycerin, which is taken by some heart patients, is thought to occasionally cause cluster headaches.

Most headaches will be tension or migraine, although almost anything can cause headaches. Doctors have long lists of various types of headaches and their causes and will be able to give you a more specific name once they find the reason for it. A medical history, physical exam, laboratory work, and specialized X rays might be used to help with the detective work of tracking down why your head is hurting.

Many patients worry that a persistent headache signals a brain tumor, but very few headaches are actually caused by tumors. Going to the doctor, though, can ease your fear if that is what you suspect.

Always go to a doctor immediately if you experience the worst headache you've ever had, if you have vision changes, trouble talking, weakness or numbness in your arms or legs, loss of balance or consciousness, if the pain wakes you up out of a deep sleep, or if you run a fever of more than 101 degrees. You should also call your doctor if a headache lasts more than four weeks.

TENSION HEADACHES
What You Can Do

Treating tension headaches is geared toward finding the cause of the headache and discovering what treatment helps. Tension headaches tend to be unpredictable, and triggers can be chemical, physical, or stress related. To make it even more difficult, the headache may develop up to twelve hours after the trigger occurred, so finding the root of the headache can take time and effort.

One of the best tools is to keep a diary of everything you eat, smell, and do and when headaches occur. Then you can look back after a week or two and see if a pattern develops. If you go away on vacation for a week or two and the headaches disappear, don't assume it was stress from the job that caused it. It could be something in your environment (such as chemical odors) or the foods you eat when you're at home that sets off the headache. You might also check with the company doctor or nurse to see if anyone else in your building is having headaches, too, because it could be something in the work environment, besides stress, that gives you a headache. Some common environmental triggers include pesticides, solvents (such as paint thinner), carbon monoxide, air systems (particularly in closed buildings where you can't open the windows), and some people claim to have developed headaches in buildings containing radon.

If nothing becomes obvious to you, begin deleting certain foods or activities that you think might trigger a headache. Always delete the suspected items one at a time for at least a week each to see if there is any change in the headaches. Food triggers can be just about anything you eat, but some that seem to cause more headaches are chocolate, nut oils, alcohol, processed meats, milk products, and artificial sweeteners. The chemicals we use to process and prolong the life of our food are also common triggers. One of the most notorious is the Chinese restaurant headache, caused by monosodium glutamate (MSG), a flavor enhancer. Glutamate is a chemical in our bodies that excites nerves, and an excited nerve is usually a painful nerve, so it may be that MSG mimics that excitement. Lots of foods besides Chinese contain MSG, especially fast food. Foods containing tyramine, a food additive, are also known to cause headaches.

Caffeine helps some headaches, especially migraines, but it can cause headaches in others. It clamps down blood vessels, decreasing blood flow, which can starve muscles and nerves, making them hurt. Some nonprescription headache remedies contain caffeine, so if it seems to make your headaches worse, check the labels of your pain relievers to make certain they don't contain caffeine.

Smoking constricts blood vessels and tenses muscles, so it makes headaches worse. Smokers often say smoking relaxes them, but it doesn't have the same effect on their bodies. Alcohol doesn't help with headaches, either, and can cause them, especially in the case of hangovers.

Stress is a leading factor in tension headaches, and for those who get one to three headaches a year, rest and nonprescription pain relievers may be the only treatment they need. If your headaches are more frequent and interfere

with your lifestyle, then it might be time to look for the
stress trigger or triggers that bring on your headaches, if
you and your doctor have eliminated other causes.

Many people get help from the numerous books on the
market teaching stress reduction and relaxation techniques.
It's sometimes difficult to see which stress is triggering
your headaches, and you might try some community classes
teaching stress reduction. There are hundreds of techniques
to reduce stress and even more people teaching such
classes, so if you try one and it doesn't work, you might
try another teacher or class. Books and classes are fairly
inexpensive ways to try to control the stress in everyday
life.

It can take weeks or months to figure out a trigger for
headaches, and sometimes you never find it, but it's worth
the time and effort to understand why you are getting headaches. Even if you can't completely eliminate the triggers,
whether they are physical or emotional, knowing what
causes them often leads to reducing the number and frequency of headaches.

If your headaches often begin at the back of the neck
and the base of the skull, exercise can strengthen and relax
the muscles there. Gently stretching your neck increases
blood flow to the area, which carries away toxins and brings
nutrients to the painful area. Exercise in general is good for
tension headaches because it releases stress, but those with
tension headaches often find themselves in a Catch-22 situation where exercise would be good for them, but the
headache makes them not want to exercise. Massage offers
some of the same advantages of exercise, increasing blood
flow and relaxing muscles. Certified massage therapists can
often teach you exercises for your neck and scalp that will
help with tension headaches.

Cold compresses, placed where the pain originates, cool
the nerves, slowing them down. Never place the ice or cold
pack directly on the skin because it can cause frostbite, so
use a washcloth or other piece of cloth to protect the skin.
Heat doesn't seem to work well for most headaches because
it doesn't penetrate as deeply as cold.

Liniments and creams can help loosen injured and

stressed muscles. Some of the creams contain capsaicin, which is derived from chili peppers, and it's not a good idea to use these creams on the temples or anywhere near the face because they could accidentally get in the eyes, nose, or mouth. Capsaicin can be used safely on the back of the neck.

Your local pharmacy probably has an entire wall of medicines for headache relief, but always check with a pharmacist or your doctor before combining nonprescription medications with each other or with prescription medicines. As long as you get the okay from a health professional, it's safe to mix and match these drugs to see what's best for you, but always follow the label directions.

Headache medications need to do two things: relieve inflammation and reduce pain. Acetaminophen (Tylenol) lessens pain, but doesn't do much for inflammation. Never take more than 3,000 milligrams a day (six extra-strength tablets). However, you can combine acetaminophen with other nonprescription medicines if you need to, but only after checking with a doctor or a pharmacist. Some brand names usually associated with aspirin, such as Bayer and Excedrin, now come in acetaminophen form, too, so always read the ingredients and make sure you aren't combining two acetaminophen brands when you think you're combining aspirin and acetaminophen.

Nonsteroidal anti-inflammatories (NSAIDs), such as ibuprofen (Advil) and naproxen (Naprosyn), should always be taken with a meal because they can irritate an empty stomach. There are many forms of NSAIDs on the market these days, and if one doesn't work for you, another one might.

Aspirin is sometimes combined with other ingredients, such as caffeine, so always read the label carefully to make certain you know just what you are taking. Never take more than 3,000 milligrams a day without first clearing it with your doctor.

All these medications have a ceiling effect, or a maximum dose that does the most good. Some patients think that if two pills are good, then four must be better, but that is not the case. Once you exceed the ceiling dose, the extra medicine is not doing your pain any good and could be harming your body. Too much acetaminophen, for example, can lead to liver damage. Taking too much medicine can also make your headaches worse. If you take too many pills too quickly, as the medicine wears off, it can actually give you another headache, called a rebound headache, which in turn causes you to take even more medicine. Always build up slowly to maximum doses and taper off slowly as you no longer need them.

Acupuncture helps some patients with headaches, as does biofeedback, which can be especially helpful with headaches caused by stress. There are lots of devices and gadgets on late-night television and in magazines that promise help with headaches, such as special pillows, electrical muscle stimulators, and massaging caps. Patients are often tempted to try unconventional treatments for headaches, but be wary of wasting time with these treatments when you could be using something that works. Always make certain you get a money-back guarantee with any unconventional treatment so you aren't wasting your money as well as your time.

What Your Doctor Can Do

A doctor's most important job is to find out what's causing your headaches and reassure you that your headaches aren't signaling something dangerous. Because headaches can be caused by anything and everything, treatments vary, depending on the type of headache and what's causing it. Individual doctors often have their own methods for dealing with chronic headaches, using what they've learned works best.

Most tension headaches aren't predictable, so doctors have to treat the symptoms once they appear. Migraines often give warning signs, so the goal of migraine treatment is to break the headache before the pain begins, but patients with tension headaches have to wait until the headache appears before they can try to stop it.

Doctors will often experiment with combinations of prescription drugs for persistent headaches, trying to find what works best for each patient. Prescription NSAIDs and salicylates (aspirin compounds) might be combined with a muscle relaxant, for example. Tricyclic antidepressants given in low doses work in the brain to restore normal sleep cycles, relaxing muscles and helping the body get the rest it needs. Narcotics are very rarely used for headaches.

Physical therapy might be prescribed to strengthen and relax tensed muscles. Sometimes, transcutaneous electrical nerve stimulators (TENS), which stimulate muscles with a mild electrical current, will be used to get more blood and nutrients to a sore muscle. Manipulation therapy, such as chiropractic care, can also be used to heal injured and tensed muscles, increasing blood flow that washes away toxins and brings in a fresh supply of nutrients to help the muscle get better.

Combining medicines and physical therapy or manipulation therapy usually helps most tension headaches, but when it doesn't, it might be time to ask to be referred to a multidisciplinary pain center, where therapies and treatments can be individualized for your particular headache. Attacking stubborn headaches with a combination of therapies and medicines often gives a better chance for relief than individual methods.

Psychologists and psychiatrists specially trained in pain treatment can teach relaxation techniques that relieve stress and also unwind tensed muscles, restoring normal blood flow and taking pressure off nerves. These techniques can also train the body to release its natural painkillers when you need them.

If doctors can identify specific nerves causing the headaches, they sometimes inject local anesthetic, blocking the pain signal and giving the nerve a chance to relax, breaking the pain cycle. These can be given on the front, sides, or back of the head, depending on which nerve is irritated.

Harriet, seventy-two, suffered tension headaches for ten years that put her life on hold when they occurred. The headaches occurred one or two times a year and lasted for several days, starting in the left side on the back of her head, traveling into the neck. Sometimes the pain sent her to the emergency room. She didn't have any nausea with these headaches, but she described the pain as sharp and traveling. Heat packs, ice packs, and lying down gave some relief, and her family doctor prescribed mild narcotics to get her through the attacks.

But on the eighteenth day of one attack, her doctor sent her to a neurologist who confirmed it was a tension headache and not something more dangerous, and sent her to a multidisciplinary pain center. At the pain center, an anesthesiologist located a nerve on the back of her head where the headaches seemed to originate and gave her a nerve block, injecting local anesthetic and a small amount of steroid into the nerve. The headache disappeared for two days, then slowly began returning, so she was injected again, and this time the headache disappeared for four months. Now she gets one or two injections a year to prevent the headaches.

Tensed muscles can also be injected with local anesthetic to break their cycle of pain. These shots are given in nerve relay stations, called trigger points, within the muscles where pain signals are concentrated.

Inflamed nerves in the neck can cause headaches and these are sometimes helped by cervical (in the vertebrae of the neck) epidurals. Epidurals inject local anesthetic and sometimes a small amount of steroid into the epidural space, the area between the ligaments of the spine and the spinal cord. This space doesn't get any blood circulation, so toxins and injuries in it have difficulty healing. By injecting the space, it washes out any toxins and allows the nerves passing through it to heal.

Margaret, fifty-eight, had a history of arthritis in her neck, pain in her jaw, and tension headaches, but after a car accident, the headaches became worse. All activities increased the pain and only heat and ice packs seemed to help. She had had three temporomandibular joint (TMJ, the hinge where the jaw joins the skull) surgeries before her accident, but none gave her much relief from the jaw pain.

The headaches were a seven on a scale of ten, with ten being the worst pain, and she described them as sharp and shooting.

Margaret's doctor prescribed muscle relaxants, NSAIDs, and tricyclic antidepressants, but when the pain didn't get any better, he gave her a mild narcotic, which helped a little. He sent her to a multidisciplinary pain center where doctors discovered her muscles were especially tight in her upper back, shoulders, neck, and jaw. An anesthesiologist tried a steroid cervical epidural, which helped relax the shoulder, back, and neck muscles, and also gave some relief to her jaw. She was given a series of three more epidurals over the course of a year, and each time she got better and better. The epidurals even helped with the jaw pain, relaxing those muscles. Now she has an epidural about once a year to keep her pain free.

Behind the nose is a group of nerves called the sphenopalatine ganglion, which supply sensation through the face and head. To treat pain, doctors used to use a very long needle to go up the nose and inject the ganglion with lidocaine, a local anesthetic; but that unpleasant experience has now been replaced with a much less painful and scary nose spray. Numbing those nerves often stops a headache, and the prescription nose spray can be administered at home without a doctor's visit and a frightening needle.

When severe headaches can't be helped by any other means and doctors can identify a specific nerve causing the headache, sometimes the nerve is killed either through radiofrequency, cryoanalgesia, or injecting it with chemicals. Radiofrequency and cryoanalgesia are described more fully in chapter 13. Occasionally, surgeons cut the nerve to stop the pain, but this technique is not used very often because the nerve usually grows back, bringing the pain with it.

MIGRAINES
What You Can Do

As many as 50 percent of migraine sufferers never go to the doctor. Some are afraid they'll be told the pain is psychological, some are afraid of finding something seriously wrong, and others think there's nothing that can be done. But medical science has made great progress in treating migraines, and there's really no reason to suffer with these debilitating headaches.

Migraines frequently have a trigger, such as a smell, a food, or certain lights, so it's a good idea to follow the routines suggested under tension headaches for locating just what's causing your pain. As with tension headaches, understanding why the pain starts is often one of the best ways to prevent it.

Patients often know when they are about to get a migraine because of the aura, the sensation that proceeds the pain. Blood vessels constrict during the aura stage, when there isn't any pain, and then dilate, filling with too much blood as the pain begins. Caffeine sometimes helps during the aura stage because it clamps down blood vessels, slowing their ability to dilate. Alcohol has the opposite effect, though, and some migraine patients avoid it altogether because it can trigger migraines. Alcohol opens up blood vessels, and that is exactly what the migraine patient doesn't need.

Nonprescription drugs aren't generally as helpful for migraines as they are for tension headaches because it's not muscles that are causing the pain, but blood vessels not pumping the right amount of blood to the brain. They can dull the pain, though, and should be tried, especially the ones containing caffeine, such as Excedrin. Sometimes, though, taking nonprescription NSAIDs on a regular basis can help prevent migraines, and one study suggests aspirin can have the same effect. Never take more than the dose recommended on the bottle, though, without checking with your doctor.

Relaxation techniques learned from books or health care professionals help some people with migraine pain, too, and might even lessen attacks. Placing ice on the back of the head and neck reduces blood flow in some patients, while others report acupuncture helps them manage the pain.

What Your Doctor Can Do

The first thing a doctor needs to do is diagnose your type of headache and try to find the trigger to prevent future headaches. Headaches can be scary, so knowing what kind they are and what's causing them can be a big relief for patients.

Preventing migraines in the first place can sometimes be accomplished by taking medicines on a regular basis. Beta blockers and calcium channel blockers, which were originally designed to treat high blood pressure, can prevent blood vessels from constricting so they don't trigger a migraine. Calcium channel blockers prevent migraines, but in some patients they can cause another type of headache, so you might be switching one kind of pain for another.

Tricyclic antidepressants are sometimes given to patients to help them get a good night's sleep, which can prevent some migraines. Stress can be one of the triggers for these headaches, and getting enough sleep can lessen stress, especially getting the kind of sleep that goes through the normal sleep cycles.

For stopping a migraine once it begins, many patients today are using sumatriptan, which can be given at home by shot or in pill form. Given during the aura, or the beginning of a headache, 50 percent of patients can break the migraine before it really begins. This drug works in the brain to prevent the blood vessels from dilating and causing pain. Some patients, especially those with uncontrolled high blood pressure and severe heart disease, can't take sumatriptan, though.

Another group of drugs for breaking migraines are the ergot alkaloids, which help prevent blood vessel spasms. These drugs can be given as pills, suppositories, or shots, or in the vein in an emergency room or doctor's office. These drugs tend to cause severe nausea and sometimes different kinds of headaches, so patients sometimes feel they're just trading one problem for another. Combining ergot alkaloids with a small amount of caffeine, codeine (a narcotic painkiller), and barbiturates (which help you sleep) keeps you sleepy but can stop a migraine for some people.

Dihydroergotamines (DHE), a form of ergot alkaloid, have fewer side effects than their cousins, and some patients report this drug prevents migraines when given on a regular basis, although no scientific studies support this. These drugs are usually given as a nasal spray or as a shot you can give yourself.

Some antiseizure medications, such as valproic acid, are used for both the prevention and treatment of migraines. It's not clear exactly how these drugs work, but they might suppress the part of the brain that triggers these headaches.

Low doses of the high blood pressure medicine clonidine have reportedly helped some patients, but not enough medical studies have been done to confirm this.

Lidocaine, a local anesthetic, sprayed up the nose works for some migraines, just as it does for some tension headaches. It calms a group of nerves behind the nose that control pain throughout the head, stopping or lessening migraines.

Phenothiazines, which were originally developed to help psychotic patients, stop migraines for some people. They make you very sleepy, though, so they can't be taken if you need to function normally.

Monoamine oxidase (MAO) inhibitors were originally developed to treat high blood pressure and depression but can work for migraine patients who don't respond to any other medicines. These drugs are very dangerous, though, and can lead to uncontrolled high blood pressure and even death if you don't follow your doctor's instructions completely. Any food containing the food additive tyramine has to be avoided when taking this medication, and your doctor will give you a complete list of foods to watch for if you are placed on this drug. These drugs also interact with narcotics, and you should never take them with MAO inhibitors.

If doctors determine the migraine is triggered by a specific nerve irritating the blood vessels, they might try to block it using some local anesthetic. They don't kill the nerve, just inject it to break the cycle of pain and let it calm down.

Some migraines begin in the neck, and a cervical (in the neck vertebrae) epidural might clean the epidural space and let the blood vessels passing through it return to normal. The epidural space runs along the spinal cord between the ligaments that hold the spine together and the cord itself. By injecting local anesthetics and perhaps a small amount of steroids into the space, it reduces inflammation, allowing the area to heal on its own.

CLUSTER HEADACHES
What You Can Do

Most people with cluster headaches see a doctor right away because the pain is so intense. As with other types of headaches, finding the trigger is the biggest step in preventing them. With cluster headaches, the number one trigger is alcohol, so quitting drinking is often the best thing you can do. You may have additional triggers, so take the steps listed under tension headaches to eliminate any foods, chemicals, allergies, lights, or smells that might be helping to cause these headaches.

What Your Doctor Can Do

Cluster headaches cause short bursts of intense pain, and they are often over before painkillers can take effect, so doctors work to prevent these headaches before they begin. Doctors still don't know whether cluster headaches begin in the muscles, nerves, or blood vessels, or even if they originate inside the brain or begin in some other part of the head.

Methysergide works in the brain, blocking the nerves aggravated by cluster headaches, and successfully prevents them in about 75 percent of patients taking these pills. This drug can't be taken continuously, though, because it forms scar tissue around internal organs, so it is usually taken for a few months at a time, then discontinued for a while.

Corticosteroids are also up to 75 percent effective, although scientists aren't exactly sure how they work. Patients using this treatment are given large doses of the corticosteroids at first, then the drug is tapered off over two weeks.

When these other two drugs aren't working, doctors will sometimes try lithium, an antidepressant, that seems to help with some tough cases. Taking this drug should be managed by a headache specialist, such as a neurologist.

Once a cluster headache strikes, patients are given 100 percent oxygen to breathe for ten or fifteen minutes. The air around us has about 21 percent oxygen, so breathing the bottled oxygen gives you about five times the normal amount. Bottles of oxygen can be kept at home for treatment when a headache strikes.

Many people are used to annoying tension headaches occurring a few times a year and manage them with some nonprescription drugs and rest. But if you notice a change in the pattern of your headaches or if you develop any of the warning signs listed above, you should go see your doctor. There are lots of different types of headaches and lots of treatments, so instead of worrying about what your headaches might mean, go see a doctor and get some answers and some help.

FACE PAIN

Face pain and headaches are often related and there can be different symptoms for the same problem. Diseases and injuries of the nerves, blood vessels, and muscles of the head can trigger face pain, just as they can cause headaches. Dental, jaw, and sinus problems can cause face pain as well as headaches, so the doctor has to be a detective for face pain, too.

Most face pain involves the trigeminal nerve, which controls sensation to much of the face and some muscles used for chewing. Face pain doesn't necessarily mean there's something wrong with the trigeminal nerve, it just means it is picking up pain signals and relaying them to the brain. Trigeminal nerve pain is called trigeminal neuralgia, or tic douloureux (which means painful tic in French), and occurs most frequently in women from ages fifty to seventy. The trigeminal nerve branches throughout the face, and it is the middle third, which extends over the cheeks, that most often causes pain, although the jaw area and the upper face can also experience neuralgia. This syndrome occurs because blood vessels in the brain dilate for no known reason, pressing on the nerve where it originates. Postherpetic neuralgia, an advanced form of shingles, can also trigger trigeminal neuralgia as the virus runs along the facial nerve. Symptoms include sharp, jabbing pain that comes and goes on one side of the face, and it can be triggered by chewing food or touching the face. The pain often appears and disappears for no known reason.

There's no medical test to determine if you have trigeminal neuralgia, although doctors can inject local anesthetic into the nerve to see if that helps with the pain, giving a pretty good clue if the pain goes away. A good patient history and physical can also lead to the diagnosis.

Treatment for trigeminal neuralgia usually includes antiseizure medicines, which alter the way the nerves send pain signals. Carbamazepine is used most often, and sometimes it is combined with baclofen or phenytoin, both antiseizure medicines, to get better results. A new antiseizure medication, gabapentin, seems to work well, but there are no clinical studies to prove it.

If the medications don't work, doctors might decide to destroy the nerve where it comes out of the brain and into the face. Sometimes chemicals are injected into the nerve to kill it, and sometimes radiofrequency, which uses heat, is used, although this method seems to cause the highest amount of loss of sensation in the face. Doctors can also insert a balloon in the hole in the skull where the nerve enters the face, inflating it to crush the nerve. All of these methods can cause some loss of sensation in the face, but not a total loss.

Correcting the problem at its root is another option if the pain can't be controlled any other way. Neurosurgeons, who are specially trained in the brain and nervous system, can perform major surgery, locating the trigeminal nerve in the brain and moving the blood vessels that push on it. This method is about 90 percent effective.

Another common cause of face pain and headaches is problems with the temporomandibular joint (TMJ), the hinge that links the jaw with the rest of the skull. This joint is rarely still, even in sleep, working constantly while you talk, eat, or even stand around. Try holding the jaw still for any length of time and you'll realize just how much it works.

Because it works hard, any pain is noticed right away and noticed a lot. TMJ disease often occurs when there's nothing wrong with the joint itself, but rather it is the muscles in the jaw that spasm. The muscles can tense from stress, or they might be injured, leading to pain in the joint like a tight rubber band pulling on the nerves. Clenching your jaw or grinding your teeth at night, both symptoms of stress, can also cause pain.

Sometimes, though, the joint simply wears out from use, injury, or because it wasn't formed correctly in the first place. This hinge joint contains a pad of dense, fibrous tissue called the meniscus that keeps the bones from knocking against each other. The meniscus in the jaw joint is thick to cushion the bones, but it can still wear out or slip out of place, causing bone to hit against bone. A worn or slipped meniscus can lead to popping and clicking in the joint and the inability to move the joint as much as you used to. Patients sometimes think the bones in the joint are deformed when they hear these noises, but the bone itself is fine, it's simply missing the correct padding.

Dentists usually diagnose TMJ disease through X rays and an exam of the teeth and tongue. They might refer you to a TMJ specialist, usually a specially trained dentist or an oral surgeon, who could order further tests, such as magnetic resonance imaging (MRI), an X ray that gives a more detailed picture of the meniscus.

One of the most common causes of TMJ disease is clenching or grinding the teeth at night. This extra stress on the joint can wear out the meniscus and tense muscles, never giving the joint a chance to relax. Your dentist will be able to tell if you're a clencher by looking at the wear pattern on your teeth and the impressions left by your teeth on your tongue.

Because TMJ is often caused by stressed muscles, anything that helps you relax those muscles can help with the pain. Massaging your jaw joints, biofeedback, and relaxation techniques can all help calm tensed muscles. It is also important to not crunch hard foods, such as hard candy and ice, and avoid chewing gum.

Clenching teeth at night can often be helped by wearing a splint, which is a piece of plastic worn on the lower teeth that helps prevent them from grinding against each other. Drugstores sell nonprescription plastic forms that you can mold to fit your teeth, but if those don't work, you might need a custom splint created by your dentist for your individual mouth.

Physical therapy may also help, as it gets more blood and nutrients to the constricted area, relaxing muscles and washing away toxins that have built up from too much tension. Psychological techniques that teach relaxation can help you consciously relax those muscles, teaching you to see just how and when you tense your jaw.

Prescription and nonprescription NSAIDs can help with the pain of TMJ, while muscle relaxants help tensed muscles learn to unwind. Tricyclic antidepressants at bedtime might be used to help you sleep better, because rested muscles tend to relax. Doctors might inject the tightened muscles with local anesthetic and a small amount of steroids to release the tension in the muscle.

Most TMJ patients don't need surgery, although an oral surgeon might perform arthroscopic surgery, where fiber optics on the end of a tube are inserted into the joint through a small slit in the skin. This procedure allows the surgeon to see if there's any damage to the joint, meniscus, or cartilage. Minor damage to the joint can also be repaired with anthroscopic surgery. Replacing a missing or deteriorated meniscus is a controversial surgery. Menisci created from man-made materials have been tried, but they actually make the problem worse, so they are no longer implanted. Oral surgeons have also tried using cartilage from ears and ribs, but it wears out too quickly to justify the surgery needed to implant them. Surgeons can do total joint replacement, like the ones done for arthritis, but this is reserved for only the most damaged joints.

Sinuses can also be responsible for face pain and headaches. Sinuses regulate the pressure in your face, making certain the ears and nasal cavities have the correct amount of air. The sinuses lie on either side of the nose and across the forehead, the lining rich with sensory fibers, so changes in pressure can cause face pain and headaches.

Allergies or infections can block off the sinuses, building pressure and pain, and treating this involves treating the cause. If it's allergies, medications that calm the allergic reaction will take care of the pain most of the time. Infections, which must be diagnosed by a doctor, might need a course of antibiotics to kill the bacteria causing the inflammation. Sometimes, surgeons go into the sinuses, making more room to relieve pressure. In both cases, over-the-counter medicines containing NSAIDs, acetaminophen, or aspirin might relieve the pain until the cause has been treated.

Atypical face pain is the term doctors use when they can't find a physical reason for the pain. There are a lot of nerves in the face that carry pain signals, which means there are a lot of things that can go wrong. Where the pain is and the type of pain will dictate how your doctor treats it. Even though doctors don't always understand why we get headaches and face pain, new technologies and medicines are creating more treatments for this elusive syndrome.

CHAPTER 9
NECK PAIN

The greatest evil is physical pain.

Saint Augustine

"A PAIN IN the neck" peppers modern conversation because neck pain plagues modern man. The neck is responsible for holding up the head, a fifteen-pound ball of muscle, skull, and brain that is often twisting, turning, and straining the muscles, bones, and nerves that run through the narrow tunnel of the neck as it struggles to keep the head balanced and secure.

Human necks contain the top seven vertebrae of the spine, called the cervical spine. Looking down on a vertebra, it looks like a human stick figure without the legs. The spinal cord runs through the chest portion, protected by the rest of the figure. The part that would be the stick figure's head is called the body, and it projects toward your front. The arms, called the transverse process, protect the nerves as they leave the spinal cord. The spinous process is the long piece that sticks toward your back, and is the part you feel when you run your fingers down your spine. Facet joints hold the vertebrae upright, allowing them to rotate so we can move our necks. They also keep the vertebrae from rubbing against each other and support the neck.

The top two vertebrae are shaped a little differently because that is where the skull connects to the spine. These vertebrae allow the head to turn, the skull swiveling on a ball joint, and they rest up under the skull, protecting this weak spot in the body.

Discs, which are about three-eighths of an inch thick, serve as cushions between the vertebrae, keeping the bones from grinding against each other. A tough outer membrane covers each disc, and a gelatinlike material, called nucleous pulposus, is inside. A herniated disc occurs when this gelatinous material leaks out, flattening the cushion. Sometimes discs don't rupture, but bulge, like a weak spot on the side of a tire. Nerves run next to the discs, so changes in the disc can pinch nerves.

Strap muscles encircle the neck, preventing it from spinning completely around. These muscles look just like straps, and they run in all different directions, stabilizing the neck and permitting fine movements, such as nodding. Larger muscles balance the head and neck and control bigger movements, such as putting your chin to your chest.

All nerves to the arms and hands originate in the cervical spine and pass through the neck muscles. The muscles in the upper arm and shoulder interconnect with those in the neck, so lifting increases the stress on the discs and muscles. We often think of lifting hurting the lower and middle back, but it can damage the neck as well.

Lots of things can hurt the neck, including sleeping in an awkward position, especially trying to sleep sitting up in an airplane or car. But playing with the kids, snapping the head around to watch a ball zip past, lifting, and almost any movement involving the head or the arms can throw it off balance, causing pain. Neck pain can be bone, muscle, or nerve pain, depending on the injury and on how the body has tried to correct it.

Like back pain, neck pain can be broken down into two categories: specific and nonspecific. Specific pain comes from a specific cause, something the health care practitioner can see on a medical test or during a physical examination, and is usually nerve or bone pain. Nonspecific pain occurs when the doctor can't find the specific cause of the pain, and is usually muscle pain in the form of a sprain or a strain.

NONSPECIFIC PAIN

Whiplash is the most common form of neck pain. It is caused when the head is thrown forward or back from a sudden stop or start, and the muscles tighten to hold the head in place. This tension and overstretching damages the muscles, causing them to swell as the body tries to heal them. Most of the time, the body does its job, and the neck hurts for a few days or weeks and then returns to normal. But if the neck has been stretched too much, individual muscle cells might break, releasing chemicals that irritate the surrounding muscle. The irritated muscles contract, decreasing blood supply to the injured area and setting up a cycle of chronic pain because the area never seems to get enough blood, which supplies oxygen and nutrients needed for healing.

Whiplash (it gets its name from the neck snapping like a whip) has become the stuff of cartoons and jokes today, with the stereotype image of someone crawling out of their car after a wreck, hand clasped to their neck. Like most stereotypes, it has some basis in truth. Many people in car accidents do get whiplash, but for most, the injured muscles return to normal within four weeks, healing on their own.

As the neck snaps, it stresses the ligaments as well as the muscles. Ligaments hold bones in place and have a lot of nerve fibers, so they hurt a lot when injured. Swollen and injured ligaments can shift the balance of the vertebrae, pulling them out of alignment. Injured muscles can do the same thing, tightening until the normal curvature of the neck is distorted. Whiplash can also cause a herniated disc in the neck, but that can be detected with special tests and then becomes specific neck pain.

Neck muscles can also be injured by using them too much: the weekend warrior syndrome, where you play basketball for three hours after not having played for ten years, or you spend all day working in the garden on the first warm day of spring.

Muscle disorders can trigger neck pain, also. Myofascial pain usually follows an injury and occurs when the muscle stays tight instead of healing and relaxing. The tightened muscle keeps blood from circulating freely to the spot and stretches nerves passing through the muscle, setting up a cycle of chronic pain.

Fibromyalgia can cause neck pain and has been described by doctors for centuries, but still, no one knows what causes it. In this disease, the muscles have aches and pains for no known reason, causing chronic pain in muscles that haven't been injured.

What You Can Do

Most neck pain will heal on its own in four to six weeks, but if you have any warning signs, see a doctor immediately. Warning signs include weakness, loss of consciousness, problems seeing, numbness or tingling in the hands and arms, pain that feels like an electrical shock, a fever of more than 101 degrees, incontinence in the bowels or bladder, and hands that turn cold and blue. These could signal more serious causes of pain and should be checked right away.

Any time the pain prevents you from enjoying a normal lifestyle, you should see a doctor. Even if it is a muscle strain or sprain that will heal gradually on its own, that doesn't mean the symptoms shouldn't be treated so your life can continue.

To prevent neck pain from beginning in the first place, gradually try new movements and activities, letting the muscles get used to the change. Healthy, strong muscles don't injure as quickly or as much as ones on couch potatoes, so exercising regularly can help prevent an injury. Any exercise utilizing the back and arms strengthens the neck.

Adjusting your work environment may help with neck

pain. Most work stations are designed for those with average heights, and if you are shorter or taller than normal, you may need to adjust your chair or your equipment to make certain you're not putting too much strain on your neck. Anyone who uses the phone a lot and has neck pain should consider getting a headset that doesn't require you to bend your neck to hold the phone in place. Squeezing those muscles and nerves to one side all the time puts too much stress on them, causing pain.

If you're waking up in the morning with neck pain, you might consider changing your pillow or mattress. Don't go charging out to spend a lot of money on new mattresses and pillows unless they have a guarantee that you can return them in thirty days and get your money back if they don't work. Pillows come in all shapes and sizes, and experimenting with various kinds might ease neck pain caused from sleeping in a position that stresses the neck.

The neck has enough to do without carrying around a lot of extra pounds, so keeping to a normal weight is one of the best things you can do for it. Fat strains muscles, bones, and nerves, weakening the body and the entire system.

Hot and cold packs can ease neck pain, helping muscles relax and easing swelling. Be careful, though, to not get the skin too hot or cold, causing another injury to the area. Never place ice directly on the skin because it can cause frostbite to an already painful area.

Over-the-counter pain medications often work for muscle neck pain. Nonsteroidal anti-inflammatories (NSAIDs) and aspirin reduce inflammation as well as easing pain. Acetaminophen reduces pain, but doesn't help with inflammation, and can be used with NSAIDs and aspirin. Talk with your doctor or pharmacist about possible interactions with any prescription or nonprescription medications you are taking already.

Liniments designed to relax muscles and dull pain can be bought in pharmacies and drugstores. A pharmacist can give advice on which ones might be best for your pain. Some creams contain salicylates, an aspirin compound, or other medicines designed to bring blood to the sore area, while others have capsaicin, derived from chili plants. Wash your hands thoroughly after applying capsaicin cream because it can burn if it gets on sensitive skin or in the eyes. Capsaicin will burn a little when it is applied. If the burning is too uncomfortable, soak a paper towel in milk and apply it to the area.

Anyone who watches a lot of late-night television knows there are lots of devices available that swear they will cure your neck pain. Some give a small current of electricity to sore muscles, and some use rollers to ease painful muscles. Sometimes they do work, but remember that most neck pain will be gone in four weeks, anyway, so it's tough to know if the device helped or if the body healed itself. Approach each of these devices with skepticism, and if you are thinking about ordering something, ask your doctor to make certain there's no chance the device will do more harm than good. Always make sure these devices come with a money-back guarantee so you won't be wasting money if they don't work.

Acupressure, where pressure is applied to tight muscles, can help with some neck pain. Charlotte, forty-two, sustained whiplash in a car accident, which left her with a sore neck and shoulders. A doctor taught her husband to do acupressure, using his thumb to press steadily and hard on certain muscle points of her neck for a few moments, then slowly releasing the pressure. Two years later, whenever the muscles flare up, he does acupressure and the pain slowly dissolves.

Massage, which gets blood and nutrients to the site and relaxes tight muscles, works for some people, as do simple stretching exercises. Avoid sharp, quick movements, but gentle stretching often helps the muscles heal. Library books or your doctor will have some suggestions.

Any healing requires a balanced diet so the body can obtain the nutrients it needs. Fresh fruits and vegetables, as well as grains, help the body obtain trace minerals and vitamins. Magnesium and calcium supplements help the muscles relax and decrease spasms.

As with all kinds of pain, alcohol, cigarettes, and caffeine slow the healing process. All deprive the body of nutrients and oxygen, interfering as it tries to repair the problem and increasing pain.

What Your Doctor Can Do

Any time neck pain lasts longer than four weeks, you should see your doctor. After an examination and maybe some tests, the doctor might have a diagnosis, which means you have specific neck pain, or he might decide your muscles are the culprits. Physical therapy is often used to retrain stubborn muscles, allowing more blood and nutrients in so your neck can heal.

Manipulation therapy, used by chiropractors and doctors of osteopathy (DOs), works for some patients. Manipulation serves much the same purpose as physical therapy, working the muscles so they relax and quit spasming, letting in a fresh blood supply that carries nutrients and washes out toxins. Manipulation therapy also can help the ligaments relax, allowing the cervical spine to return to its normal position.

Injection therapy might be needed if the muscles are too sore to allow physical or manipulation therapy. An anesthesiologist injects local anesthetic into specific sites in the sore muscles, called trigger points, helping them relax and breaking the cycle of pain. Once the muscles relax, blood supply is improved and the body can better heal the area.

Some patients report help from acupuncture, which uses needles to redirect the electrical currents in the body, although there is no scientific evidence that this works. Biofeedback and relaxation therapy can help redirect the mind so it doesn't focus on the pain as much.

Medications for nonspecific neck pain include NSAIDs, both prescription and nonprescription, as well as other pain relievers. Muscle relaxants are often combined with stretching exercises to release the tension in the muscles, allowing healing nutrients and oxygen to the area.

Transcutaneous electrical nerve stimulators (TENS) use

pads placed on the skin to deliver a small amount of electricity to the muscles, disrupting the pain signal. These are generally used only in persistent muscle pain, and are discussed more fully in chapter 13.

SPECIFIC NECK PAIN

Once your doctor runs tests and determines the cause of your neck pain, then it is specific neck pain, pain that has a name. Herniated discs, arthritis, infection, osteoporosis, compression fractures (where weakened bone is broken just by normal stresses), cancer, and spinal stenosis (where the opening for a nerve running out of the spinal column is too small, pinching it) are just some of the more common causes of specific neck pain.

Specific neck pain is pain that shows up on medical tests, such as X rays, magnetic resonance imaging (MRI), computerized tomography (CT scans), blood work, nerve tests, bone scans, and physical examinations. Specific neck pain has a name, a definite physical finding, that tells the doctor and the patient what's happening in the neck.

What You Can Do

Any time you have any of the warning signs, go see your doctor immediately. Warning signs include weakness, loss of consciousness, difficulty seeing, numbness or tingling in the hands and arms, pain that feels like an electrical shock, a fever of more than 101 degrees, incontinence in the bowels and bladder, and hands that turn cold and blue. Any time the pain is interfering with your normal lifestyle or if it lasts longer than four weeks, you should go see a doctor.

The techniques and methods listed in What You Can Do under Nonspecific Neck Pain also work for specific neck pain.

What Your Doctor Can Do

The first thing the doctor will do is try to find out what is causing the pain. After a physical examination, medical history, and perhaps some tests, he'll have a better idea of the problem and can begin to chart a course of treatment.

Physical therapy is often prescribed for neck pain because it accomplishes so much. Strengthening the neck and its muscles and ligaments lets fresh blood into the injured area, which carries away toxins and helps the neck to heal. Because ligaments are what hold the bones in place, getting them in shape can help the vertebrae align better and take pressure off nerves.

Chiropractic care and manipulation therapy can sometimes accomplish the same goals as physical therapy by creating strong neck muscles and ligaments, allowing bones to return to their normal alignment. Physical therapy might be combined with chiropractic care or manipulation therapy, with both working in their individual ways to increase blood flow and healing.

Six sessions of chiropractic care, manipulation therapy, or physical therapy should be enough to notice some improvement. The pain may not be much better in those six sessions, but if you can tell you are stronger or that your neck is able to move better, that counts as improvement. If after six sessions, there is no improvement or the pain is worse, it's time to talk to your doctor to see if maybe some other treatment should be tried.

Sometimes patients need psychological help to deal with the pain and to teach them relaxation techniques. Pain is debilitating to the mind as well as the body, and it can help to talk with someone about it. Hypnosis and biofeedback are sometimes used to help patients handle the psychological and physical effects of neck pain.

Medications can accomplish two goals with neck pain: reducing inflammation in the injured area and relieving pain. NSAIDs, both over-the-counter and prescription, can relieve swelling as well as provide pain relief. Other non-narcotic painkillers might be prescribed and steroids might be given to reduce swelling, but only for short periods of time. Muscle relaxants do just what their name implies, letting tensed muscles unwind. For persistent pain, doctors might turn to narcotics, but like steroids, they are usually only given for short periods because of their side effects, which are described more in chapter 12.

Injecting muscles, joints, or nerves with local anesthetic lets the site relax, and can break the pain cycle, although it frequently takes a series of shots to get the desired effect. Placing a local anesthetic, and perhaps some steroids, directly into the pain site can be helpful in restoring blood flow to the area once the tightened muscle or nerve relaxes.

Frank, eighty-eight, was raking his yard when he developed neck pain on his right side, which soon became a constant stabbing, dull, aching pain. Heat packs were the only thing that helped. He went to his internist who prescribed physical therapy. The physical therapy helped while Frank was in the office, but by the time he'd get back home, the pain returned. By this time, the pain became a nine on a scale of ten, with ten being the worst pain, and he couldn't sleep anymore.

His internist sent him to a multidisciplinary pain center where X rays showed Frank had a lot of arthritis in his neck that was affecting the discs and the facet joints (the ones that hold the vertebrae in place). An anesthesiologist prescribed NSAIDs and a mild muscle relaxant and injected two of the facet joints with local anesthetic and steroids.

Frank improved, but the pain then switched more to the left side, so he was given an MRI, which showed arthritis in facet joints on the left. The anesthesiologist gave Frank a cervical (in the neck) facet block, where steroids and a local anesthetic were injected into the diseased area. Within a week, Frank was pain free and only took nonprescription NSAIDs once in a while for flare-ups.

Shots in the muscles are called trigger points, because they are given in trigger points, which are nerve relay stations scattered throughout muscles. These spots concentrate the pain signal, and inserting a needle and medicine can sometimes reset them, letting them forget they are supposed to be tensed. Many different medicines are used in trigger points, depending on the patient and the type of pain, including local anesthetics, water, steroids, NSAIDs, or plant enzymes. Sometimes, the doctor will simply insert a needle with no medication and twist it, stimulating the body's immune response to the injured area.

Cervical nerve root injections use local anesthetics and sometimes small amounts of steroids at the base of the nerve in the spinal canal. The patient might be given a mild sedative before the injections to make him more comfortable. These nerve blocks are only used when the doctor can identify specific nerves that are causing the pain, and they only numb the irritated nerve.

Brachial plexus nerve blocks numb the entire arm and hand for as long as eight to twelve hours. It feels as if the arms and hands have fallen asleep, so you can still move them, although they might feel weak. The brachial plexus is a group of nerves in the neck that are tightly compressed in a bundle before they branch out to the arms and hands. By injecting local anesthetic, and sometimes some steroids, into this group, it relaxes the nerves, giving them a chance to reset and forget they were irritated. Often this is done so the patient can undergo physical therapy because the pain is too intense to allow it otherwise. Brachial plexus blocks are most often used for reflex sympathetic dystrophy and nerve inflammation.

Cervical epidurals help reduce swelling in the epidural space of the neck and cleanse the area of toxins released when a disc is injured. The doctor numbs the skin then injects salt water, steroids, and sometimes a local anesthetic into the epidural space of the painful vertebrae, giving the damaged area time to heal and often preventing surgery. These are used for herniated discs and pinched nerves, and to slow the advance of arthritis.

Mick, seventy-one, slowly developed pain in his arm down to his wrist, which he described as sharp, throbbing, numb, aching, and tingling. His right hand became swollen, and he tried heat and ice packs, but they didn't help. His family doctor prescribed NSAIDs, but the pain didn't get any better, so he was given mild narcotics and referred to a neurosurgeon. By this time, Mick found it difficult to write and often dropped things he held in his right hand.

The neurosurgeon diagnosed severe arthritis in Mick's neck and a disc that was pinching a nerve, and sent him to a multidisciplinary pain center. There, an anesthesiologist performed a cervical steroid epidural, which helped Mick use his hand but didn't help much with the pain. Two weeks later, a second epidural relieved all of Mick's pain and he was able to quit using his medications and regained full use of his hand.

Radiofrequency, which uses heat, is sometimes used in neck pain to kill nerves that can't be calmed any other way. Cryoanalgesia, which uses cold, also serves the same purpose. Both of these options are discussed more fully in chapter 13. Doctors can also inject chemicals, such as alcohol, into a nerve to kill it, but the nerve frequently grows back.

Often, a combination of the above techniques works better than one alone, so if your pain doesn't get better in two or three weeks using just one of these procedures, then you might want to consider getting a referral to a multidisciplinary pain center, where specialists can coordinate treatment and medications that will benefit your unique pain.

Often, the first path of treatment will not include surgery. Herniated discs, for example, only need immediate surgery in about 20 percent of cases. Medicines and therapy can take care of many neck problems.

Jerry, fifty, had been in a car accident, suffering a whiplash that X rays showed didn't involve any bone, just the muscle. Off and on for fourteen years he had neck pain that often traveled down his left arm, causing sharp pain that sometimes felt like electricity in his fingers. Jerry noticed that stress aggravated the pain, that it got worse as the day progressed, and that lifting intensified the pain. Heat packs and lying down helped, but as the years progressed, so did the pain, until he had trouble sleeping and working at his desk.

Jerry's family doctor couldn't prescribe NSAIDs for the pain because Jerry had a history of ulcers, and NSAIDs can cause stomach distress. He prescribed narcotics and muscle relaxants for the pain, but Jerry couldn't work because both medicines made him too groggy, so the family doctor referred him to a multidisciplinary pain center.

At the pain center, the doctors ordered an MRI, which diagnosed specific neck pain caused by a large, herniated disc on the left side. Jerry was referred to a surgeon, but he preferred to not have surgery, and the doctors agreed that more conservative measures could be tried first.

Jerry was placed on tricyclic antidepressants to help him sleep, and biofeedback and a TENS unit were tried, but he got no relief. He declined physical therapy because he'd tried it after his accident fourteen years before, and he felt it had made him worse. An anesthesiologist at the pain center gave him a steroid epidural, and he reported 50 percent relief and cut back on his pain medications.

After a week, the pain slowly began to come back, so a second epidural was given, and for two days after the second epidural, he had no pain, and then he experienced 75 percent relief in his neck pain. Two weeks later, a third epidural was given, and within a month, Jerry was 90 percent better, experiencing only occasional tingling in his arm. He quit taking all his pain medications and resumed a full workload.

Because there is no blood supply in the epidural space, the body has trouble healing any injuries in that area. The white blood cells arrive to clean up the injury, but there's no way for them to be washed away. No one knows exactly how the epidural works, but the theory is that injecting medications into the space washes out any debris and the steroids help reduce swelling, giving the body a chance to heal itself.

If you have specific neck pain, then you have a diagnosis of what's causing the pain. Before you consent to surgery, make sure you understand exactly what is wrong and how this surgery can repair it. Don't be afraid to get a second opinion and get references for your surgeon. Both orthopedic surgeons, who are trained in bone surgery, and neurosurgeons, who study the nerves, do neck surgery, and you'll be referred to the correct type, depending on your injury.

Louise, seventy-two, gradually developed neck pain that radiated down both her arms and up the back of her head, until it was bad enough that she went to see her internist, who ordered X rays that showed she had arthritis. She was referred to an orthopedic surgeon who injected cortisone (a steroid) in her shoulders, but that didn't help. Her internist then sent her to physical therapy, which helped some, as did NSAIDs, muscle relaxants, and a mild narcotic. She also tried chiropractic care and a TENS unit, but those didn't help much, either.

Louise was sent to a multidisciplinary pain center where she was given tricyclic antidepressants to help her sleep, capsaicin cream, and a series of three epidurals. She began feeling better, but two weeks later, the pain came back. She was referred to a neurosurgeon who ordered an MRI, which indicated she needed surgery because nerves were being pinched where the opening for them was too small (spinal stenosis). The surgery worked well for the pain in her arms and the back of her head but didn't help much for the pain in her neck, so she was sent back to the pain center.

An anesthesiologist at the pain center gave her a series of trigger point injections for the muscle spasms and also injected her facet joints with local anesthetic and a small amount of steroid. The pain slowly got better, and Louise returned to her normal routine.

Another way to take pressure off neck nerves is an anterior cervical fusion. *Anterior* refers to the front of the body, and *cervical* means the neck vertebrae. For this operation, which has an 80 to 90 percent success rate, the surgeon sometimes removes the damaged disc or he might also put in a piece of bone or a screw to hold the vertebrae apart so they don't crunch together. If bone is used it is usually taken from the patient's pelvic bone or from a cadaver.

In thoracic outlet syndrome, a rib or the anterior scalene muscle (the muscle covering the area from the collarbone to the first rib) is putting pressure on the nerves and causing pain. In these cases, surgeons can remove ribs, whether it is an extra one or the first rib, to take pressure off the nerves in the neck. If the ribs aren't the problem, surgeons can also remove the anterior scalene muscle so it won't tighten nerves and cause pain.

When conservative treatments and surgery fail, doctors sometimes use spinal cord stimulators (SCSs) to block the pain signal. These devices place electrodes next to the spinal cord and use electricity to derail pain signals. They are generally used as a last resort and only in carefully selected patients.

Intrathecal pumps might be tried if an SCS has failed, but studies haven't shown yet whether they are effective in the long term. But this technology and the medicine used in it, is changing all the time, improving effectiveness and decreasing side effects. Both pumps and SCSs are discussed more fully in chapter 13.

Your neck has a difficult job to do and a lot of possibilities for things to go wrong, so it's no wonder so many of us get neck pain from time to time. Remember that most neck pain will heal itself in four weeks, but if yours persists, there are lots options and treatments so you don't have to literally live with a pain in the neck.

CHAPTER 10
MORE PAIN SYNDROMES

I wish no living thing to suffer pain.

Percy Bysshe Shelley

FIBROMYALGIA

THE MUSCLE ACHES and pains of fibromyalgia have been described for hundreds of years, but there are still some doctors today who believe it doesn't exist. It wasn't until 1990 that modern medicine established formal written criteria for this disease. No tests exist to confirm a diagnosis of fibromyalgia, and all tests, including biopsies of the sore muscles, appear normal, yet somewhere between 1 and 2 percent of the population of the United States suffers from the constant aching of this disease.

Fibromyalgia is characterized by widespread, diffuse muscle pain that lasts more than three months. It's an all-over aching that just doesn't go away, and no one knows why. These patients often have fatigue, sleep disturbances, and morning stiffness. Women get this disease ten times more often than men. Seventy-five percent of patients with chronic fatigue syndrome have fibromyalgia, but the reverse is not true.

Fibromyalgia is often associated with other diseases, although doctors aren't sure why. Forty percent of fibromyalgia patients have osteoarthritis, 25 percent have rheumatoid arthritis, and about a third have irritable bowel syndrome.

Studies have shown that a lack of sleep may cause fibromyalgia or make it worse. In one study, college students who were deliberately deprived of sleep developed symptoms of fibromyalgia, which then disappeared when they were allowed to resume their normal sleep patterns. It's important for anyone with this disease to develop restful sleep patterns that allow for all the cycles of normal sleep.

What You Can Do

The two most important things for the fibromyalgia patient are to get enough sleep and to exercise. Because they are in pain, fibromyalgia patients tend to not want to exercise, but it is better to keep their muscles strong, and patients report that regular exercise does make them feel better, and it can lead to better sleep.

Almost any kind of exercise is good for the fibromyalgia patient, but make certain you exercise all the major muscle groups. If you bicycle, walk, or run, for example, then do weights or something else for the upper body. Aerobic exercise, swimming, rowing machines, and cross-country skiing machines are good because they use muscles in the arms and legs.

Getting enough sleep and getting the right kind of sleep is essential for the fibromyalgia patient, but taking over-the-counter sleep medications is not the answer. Most of these medicines are not intended for long-term use because they don't allow normal sleep patterns. Melatonin helps some patients sleep better, and the antihistamine diphenhydramine hydrochloride (Benadryl), which helps many people to sleep, can usually be taken on a regular basis.

Some patients report taking calcium, magnesium, and zinc supplements give relief, probably because these minerals are used by the muscles. Alcohol disrupts sleep patterns, so it should be avoided by those with fibromyalgia. Smoking decreases blood flow to the muscles, which can make them hurt worse. Caffeine has the same effect, but to a lesser extent, and should only be used in moderation.

Guaifenesin, an over-the-counter medicine found in many cough syrups, seems to relieve the muscle aches and pains of some patients, although there's no scientific data to show this. Guaifenesin comes in pill form, but it can be difficult to find. Most patients take it in the form of cough syrup, but read the label carefully because you don't want to be taking guaifenesin with any other medicine in it. Most patients start with 300 milligrams twice a day and can increase the dose up to four times a day. This method can take weeks to work, so give it some time. Some doctors believe you shouldn't take any aspirin (salycilates) in either oral or cream form with guaifenesin because it can make it less effective.

Massage might make the muscles feel better, but be sure to tell your massage therapist that you have fibromyalgia and where you have tender spots.

Learning relaxation techniques can also help with the aching. Relaxed muscles don't hurt as much as tensed ones because they get better blood flow, bringing nutrients and taking away toxins released when the muscle is tensed. Relaxation might also help improve sleep.

Nonprescription medications can often give significant relief for patients, as can liniments and creams designed for sore muscles. Acetaminophen (Tylenol), aspirin, and non-steroidal anti-inflammatories (such as ibuprofen and naproxen) can all help with the pain from fibromyalgia. The liniments and creams bring blood to sore areas, helping them to relax and heal. Creams containing capsaicin, which is derived from chili peppers, need to be handled with extra care. This type of cream can burn if it gets in the eyes or on other tender tissues. Always wash your hands thoroughly after applying capsaicin cream or wear rubber gloves when you rub it in. It should feel warm, but if it is too painful, you can soak a paper towel in milk and place it on the site.

What Your Doctor Can Do

Keeping active and taking medications are the two mainstays of fibromyalgia treatment. It is very important that you keep active because if you don't use your muscles, they waste away, which makes them hurt even more. Your doctor might suggest physical therapy to teach you stretching and the right kind of exercise. Physical therapists might incorporate transcutaneous electrical nerve stimulators (TENS), which use small amounts of electricity to stimulate muscles, into your routine.

Your doctor might also prescribe a muscle stimulator, which looks like a TENS unit, but is designed to strengthen muscles, not block pain. Fibromyalgia patients need to exercise, but often don't want to because of the pain. With a muscle stimulator, pads are placed over the painful muscle groups, and electricity stimulates the muscles so they contract as if they were getting exercise.

Prescription NSAIDs help some fibromyalgia patients, and doctors often prescribe tricyclic antidepressants not only to help the patient sleep, but also to help with the pain. About a dozen forms of tricyclic antidepressants exist today, so if one isn't working for you, ask your doctor to try another. Muscle relaxants help some patients, relaxing stiff and tight muscles, but not everyone gets relief from these medicines. Some doctors are using the antiseizure medicine gabapentin, but this medication is new and no studies confirm that it helps. Doctors aren't sure why antiseizure medicines work for pain, but they speculate it disrupts the pain signal in the brain.

Patients sometimes report that their pain is worse at certain times of the month, so doctors might prescribe hormone therapy to smooth out the hormonal highs and lows. Low doses of testosterone, estrogen, or birth control pills can be used for hormone therapy.

If nothing else works, doctors might prescribe low doses of narcotics to help with the pain.

Psychologists and psychiatrists can teach relaxation therapy, hypnosis, and biofeedback that will give spasmed muscles a chance to relax. These techniques also train the body to release its own natural painkillers, called endorphins and enkephalins, sometimes allowing you to use less medicine.

Flare-ups in pain might require injections in the sore

muscles. Some doctors simply use a needle with no medication, while others inject a local anesthetic or a combination of medicines. Steroids are generally not used in these injections because studies show they aren't effective for fibromyalgia pain. These shots break the cycle of pain, resetting the muscles and giving temporary relief, but the effects don't usually last for very long.

MYOFASCIAL PAIN SYNDROME

About a fifth of those aged twenty to sixty have this muscle pain syndrome, although some estimates place the number as high as 50 percent. Myofascial pain is those chronic sore spots that come and go, usually irritated by overdoing or some new movement. For most people, these sore spots become a part of their life and usually don't interfere too much with daily routines, but some require a doctor's treatment when the areas flare up.

Myofascial pain occurs when a part of a muscle spasms, irritating nerves and tightening, which restricts blood flow to the area. Many things can trigger myofascial pain, including accidents and injuries that hurt muscles and set up a cycle of pain. These areas of pain, called trigger points, continue to hurt after the initial injury has healed, spasming and irritating nerves as the muscle falls into a routine of discomfort. For most people, four weeks is usually enough time to heal from an injury and the muscles return to their normal pattern, but in some cases, the muscle continues to spasm like a broken record. The pain can get better and then worse, coming and going sometimes for no known reason.

Myofascial pain can also accompany other injuries. For example, you can have a herniated disc and myofascial pain, or a broken bone and myofascial pain, or pain from an operation and myofascial pain. And it gets even more confusing because myofascial pain can mimic other disorders, making an arm or leg numb or tingling as if there

were nerve damage or causing a burning pain that might
be mistaken for something else.

Once myofascial pain is suspected as the culprit, it can
usually be diagnosed by pushing on specific areas, called
trigger points, that can reproduce the pain. Trigger points
are scattered all over the body, wherever there are muscles,
and they correspond closely with acupuncture points. Trigger points reproduce pain along very specific routes, and
when the doctor pushes or pinches these trigger points, the
pain will follow that path. Trigger points in the rhomboid
muscles, which lie between the shoulder blades, will cause
pain in the shoulder, for example, and the trapezius muscle,
which runs from the base of the skull and down the back,
has trigger points that cause pain in the head, face, and arm.
If a doctor pushes on a trigger point and it reproduces the
pain you've been experiencing, then he's diagnosed myofascial pain.

What You Can Do

Treatment for myofascial pain centers around relaxing the
tight muscle so it stops irritating the nerves, allowing blood
flow in the area to return to normal. One of the best ways
to help the muscle heal is to lightly stretch it, gently pulling
to encourage it to relax. You may have to wait until the
original injury has healed to begin stretching, but if you
experience whiplash, it's best to begin stretching those neck
and back muscles right away so they don't tighten up. If
you're being treated by a health care professional for whiplash, always check with him first before beginning any
stretching.

Even gentle stretching may be painful for some patients,
and it sometimes helps to place a cold compress on the sore
muscle before stretching to numb the area. Never place ice
or a cold pack directly on the skin, and check frequently
to make sure the area isn't getting so cold that it causes
frostbite.

Heat packs relax sore muscles, stimulating blood flow.

Tensed and injured muscles release toxins that irritate surrounding tissue and nerves, and increasing blood flow to the area allows the body to wash away the toxins and deliver healing nutrients.

Exercise also stimulates blood flow, bringing a fresh supply to injured muscles. There's no reason not to exercise if you have myofascial pain, but if you're being treated by a health care professional, always check with him first before beginning an exercise routine.

Massage and acupressure, which involves pushing on the trigger points, also bring more blood to the muscle and help relax it. If it's a muscle you can reach, you can massage it gently to stimulate blood flow, and if you decide on a professional massage therapist, be sure to tell him which muscle is causing you trouble.

Smoking restricts blood flow and the muscle needs more blood, not less. Too much caffeine has the same effect, as does alcohol. A diet emphasizing whole grains and fresh produce gives your body the tools it needs to heal, while taking calcium, magnesium, and zinc supplements gives the muscles extra doses of nutrients they need.

Nonprescription pain relievers, such as NSAIDs, aspirin, and acetaminophen can help with flare-ups and might make stretching less painful. Liniments and creams designed to help sore muscles work for some people because they increase blood flow. Capsaicin cream also helps relieve pain in the muscle, but be careful when applying it. Capsaicin contains substances from chili peppers and can burn if it gets in the eyes or touches tender tissue. Wash your hands after applying it, or use rubber gloves. It burns a little when applied, but if it hurts too much, soak a paper towel in milk and apply it to the area.

Relaxation techniques you learn from books or tapes could also help with myofascial pain by releasing the tension in sore muscles. They also help you learn to relax those areas, which might help with flare-ups of pain.

Because myofascial pain is so common, there are lots of nonprescription devices to help with sore muscles. Before investing in any of these devices, be certain you have a money-back guarantee, because you can spend a lot of money on these things and not get any relief. There are devices that deliver a mild dose of electricity to the muscle, those that let you push on sore muscles or massage them, and some that stimulate the muscle through vibration. They work on the principle of increasing blood flow to the area, and they might work for you. But remember that most muscle pain will heal on its own in four weeks, so be careful before spending a lot of money.

What Your Doctor Can Do

Myofascial pain usually has a good prognosis. It may take several weeks or months of treatment, but generally doctors can turn an active trigger point into an inactive one. Additional treatments may be required if the trigger point flares again.

Doctors often inject the active trigger points to stimulate blood flow and relax the muscle, breaking the cycle of pain. Some doctors use only the needle, while others might inject a local anesthetic or a combination of medicines that releases tension in the sore spot. One trigger point might be irritating another, or the injury could be widespread, so more than one shot might be needed. Usually, a series of these injections is necessary to teach the muscle to relax, and the number of shots will depend on your doctor and your injury. Shots might be given anywhere from one to three per week over several weeks or months, depending on what your body needs. The shots might have to be repeated every few months to keep the muscle from reverting to its old habits.

After each shot, the patient is often instructed to do stretching exercises or goes to physical therapy to get the tightness out of the muscle. Sometimes, the sore area is sprayed with a cold liquid after the stretching to numb the muscle and keep the body's focus from it. Physical therapists might also use transcutaneous electrical nerve stimulators (TENS), which deliver a small amount of electricity to the trigger point, stimulating blood flow and encouraging the muscle to relax.

Prescription NSAIDs can ease pain while also helping to reduce swelling in the inflamed muscle. Muscle relaxants do just what their name says, loosening tightened muscles and perhaps breaking the spasm.

For myofascial pain originating in the back and neck, chiropractic care might be helpful because the manipulation will get more blood to the area to help with healing.

Biofeedback and relaxation techniques taught by psychologists or psychiatrists teach you how to relax the sore muscle and how to help your body stay relaxed so the injury isn't aggravated. These techniques also might help you stimulate your body's natural painkillers, helping with the pain as well as the healing.

CARPAL TUNNEL SYNDROME

Computers created a surge in this common pain syndrome, although it has existed as long as man has had wrists. Most often caused by repeating the same wrist motion over and over, it has become associated with people who spend their days keyboarding, but it can also be caused by a whole list of jobs from meat cutting to performing surgery.

Carpal tunnel syndrome can be caused by injuries to the wrist, but for most people it is classified as a repetitive stress injury (RSI), which means doing the same thing over and over, stressing the joint, and causing pain. RSIs aren't limited to carpal tunnel syndrome, but can occur in any part of the body where the same motion eventually causes damage, such as tennis elbow and runner's knee.

The carpal tunnel is a sheath of tissue in the wrist that houses the median nerve, a nerve that runs down the arm and into part of the thumb and the first three fingers. Carpal tunnel syndrome occurs when something inflames the sheath, compressing the nerve at the wrist. Using the wrist every day in the same way can create scar tissue, pulling on the nerve as the wrist moves. Most people with carpal tunnel syndrome experience pain in the wrist and hand, but the median nerve runs up the arm and into the neck, and the pain can occur any place along the nerve. Fifteen percent of patients with carpal tunnel syndrome experience pain in their neck.

Patients often report waking up at night with pain in their arm and wrist, describing the pain as sharp, shooting, aching, burning, with some itching or numbness. Flexing and extending the wrist tends to make the pain worse, and people suffering from the syndrome often have trouble opening jars and holding things like coffee cups for long periods of time.

Carpal tunnel syndrome is a symptom, but the term doesn't tell what's causing the pain. Arthritis, benign tumors, or anything else that can put pressure on the median nerve can cause carpal tunnel, so it's important to locate the cause of the pain so the symptoms can be treated. Once the patient and doctor discover what is causing the pain, carpal tunnel syndrome can often be treated conservatively without resorting to surgery.

You should seek treatment if you are having any of the symptoms of carpal tunnel because the sooner this problem is caught, the more likely you can be helped by conservative methods, such as splinting and exercise. Don't let the pain become unbearable before seeking help because the longer the problem lasts, the more it compresses the median nerve.

Any time, though, that you lose function in your hand, you should see your doctor immediately. Even if you don't have any pain, if you have trouble using your hand, go see your doctor. The longer you wait to get help, the more damage might be done.

What You Can Do

If you have a job that requires you to use your wrists in the same way all day, stop at least once an hour to rotate your wrists and move them from side to side. Try to take a break once an hour and do something else, whether it is using the copy machine or some other part of your job that will give your wrists a rest from that repetitive motion.

Make certain your work station is the most effective for your height. Most desks and chairs are designed for people of normal height, but they may put extra stress on your wrists if they don't put your equipment at the right level for you. The library has many books that show the correct position for arms and hands when keyboarding, or ask your company doctor or nurse for some information. If you work at a keyboard, soft bumpers that support the wrists might remove some of the stress.

Nonprescription medications like NSAIDs, aspirin, and acetaminophen often help with carpal tunnel, and if you are waking up in the night with pain, take them before you go to bed. Creams and liniments don't seem to help much with this syndrome because the nerve is too deep to be affected by them.

Some patients report that taking 100 milligrams of vitamin B_6 twice a day helps, but medical studies haven't shown this definitely works.

Wearing a splint on your wrist helps to keep it still and avoid aggravating the carpal tunnel. Most drugstores sell wrist splints. Check the package to get the right size for you.

Follow the directions on the package about keeping your wrist at the correct angle, and never wear the splint so tightly that your fingers don't look normal. If they turn red, white, or blue, you've tightened it too much. Your thumb should be able to move freely and you should be able to touch your index finger to your thumb when wearing the splint. Only wear the splint when you're doing what causes the pain, because wearing it all the time will cause the muscles to get weak, only making the problem worse. If you need to wear the splint all the time because it hurts when you don't, then see your doctor.

Studies show that by following these conservative treatments, about 75 percent of carpal tunnel patients report improvement if their symptoms are caused by RSI.

What Your Doctor Can Do

The first thing your doctor will want to do is determine if you have carpal tunnel syndrome and what is causing it, because you have to know where it's coming from before you can begin effective treatment. Your doctor will take a history and give you a physical, examining your wrists and probably asking you to perform a few tasks to assess the problem.

Sometimes, doctors perform EMGs (electromyograms) and NCVs (nerve conduction velocity tests) which show how your nerves are conducting signals. These two tests can pinpoint where the pain is coming from, giving your doctor a better handle on your diagnosis.

Prescription NSAIDs might help with the pain and reduce swelling. Steroids might be prescribed if rheumatoid arthritis is causing your carpal tunnel symptoms.

If a splint you bought at the drugstore isn't helping, then your doctor might prescribe a custom one that is designed specifically for your wrist and your problem. A physical therapist or an occupational therapist might be able to redesign your work area, making it more wrist-friendly. They can also teach you exercises for your wrist to help with the healing.

Doctors have started injecting local anesthetic and steroids into injured wrists, hoping to ease pain while helping the body heal the area. The long-term success of this method is still unconfirmed, with studies showing anywhere from 15 to 60 percent improvement for more than a few days or weeks.

If none of these techniques is successful, then surgery may be necessary to give the median nerve more room. This is a short surgery, lasting usually only ten to fifteen minutes, but it has anywhere from a 2 to 15 percent complication rate, so it is not something that should be done without trying other methods first.

Hand surgeons, orthopedic surgeons (who specialize in bones), neurosurgeons (who specialize in the nerves, brain, and spinal column), and some general surgeons perform this operation. Your doctor will recommend someone she feels is best for your surgical needs. Choose a doctor who has performed a lot of carpal tunnel surgeries and ask about his success rate.

Your surgeon might choose one of two ways to repair the damage to the wrist. The traditional method is to open the wrist with a scalpel and free the nerve, but some doctors are now beginning to insert an endoscope (a tube with a light and a small cutting edge at the end) through a small hole in the wrist to cut the sheath compressing the nerve. This second method is much newer and there's not as much research data supporting its use, but it avoids cutting into the wrist.

OSTEOPOROSIS

Osteoporosis weakens bones as it leaches out calcium, preventing them from rebuilding. We replace our entire skeleton every twenty years, but sometimes our bones don't rebuild themselves as quickly as they break down, and the bones become thinner and weaker, increasing the chance of fractures. Osteoporosis costs more than seven billion health care dollars each year, with up to a million women developing fractures in their weakened bones.

Osteoporosis is associated with postmenopausal women, but 20 percent of men over sixty-five suffer from it, too. Scientists speculate it is the lack of hormones that somehow prevents the body from continuing to build bones, and recent studies suggest that women who take replacement hormones have a decreased risk of developing osteoporosis. Other things cause it, too, though, including malnutrition, certain diseases, and some drugs, especially steroids. Not moving enough can weaken bone also, because movement stimulates bone growth.

Most osteoporosis patients don't know they have the disease until they begin to have pain, and 90 percent first go to their doctor because of pain. Low back pain is the first symptom of most of these patients, because the disease seems to weaken vertebrae first.

As the bones weaken, they can collapse, pinching nerves and compressing the spine. Compression fractures, caused when the individual vertebrae begin collapsing because they've become too thin to support the body, can cause extreme pain as nerves in the spinal column are suddenly moved and pinched.

What You Can Do

Women should take calcium and vitamin D supplements throughout their lives to keep their bones strong. It won't do you any good to take just calcium, because the body needs vitamin D to break down calcium and absorb it.

Exercise is essential in preventing osteoporosis because exercise stimulates bone growth. This doesn't mean you have to be a marathon runner your whole life, but it does mean you should exercise regularly to keep bones as strong as possible. Exercise may not completely prevent osteoporosis, but it can prevent severe cases.

It's never too late to begin either taking supplements or exercising, although if you've already developed osteoporosis, check with your doctor before beginning any exercise routine. The sooner you begin, though, the better your bones will be prepared as the body slows bone production after menopause.

What Your Doctor Can Do

If your doctor suspects osteoporosis, he can order a special X ray that detects bone density. Regular X rays can spot advanced stages of the disease, but don't show it in the early stage. If you're having back pain, your doctor might order an MRI or a CAT scan, both specialized X rays that give detailed views of the body, and these tests will also pick up any osteoporosis.

Replacement hormone therapy for women after menopause seems to help some from developing osteoporosis, or at least not as severe a case as women who don't take hormones. Not every woman can take hormones, though, and you and your doctor must decide if replacement therapy is appropriate for you.

Both men and women can take two recent drugs that can prevent osteoporosis and can help bones grow stronger once the disease is present. Aleneronate sodium (Fosamax) comes in pill form, while calcitonin was originally given as a shot, but now comes also as a nasal spray. Calcitonin can't be absorbed through the stomach because it breaks down the drug before it can do any good. You must take calcium and vitamin D with both these drugs because they simply help the body rebuild the bones, and it needs the correct building blocks.

Physical therapy and rehabilitation therapy can teach you exercises to help your bones become stronger and provide new methods to deal with a body that has weakened bones. Some patients, for example, develop a curved spine from this disease and rehabilitation therapists can help them adjust.

Sometimes doctors will prescribe a back brace to help with weakened vertebrae, but never wear one unless your doctor tells you to. By keeping the back from moving, these braces can actually encourage further deterioration of the vertebrae.

If you have back pain from osteoporosis or a compression fracture, chapter 3 details techniques and medications to help with low back pain. Compression fractures rarely need surgery because surgery can't make the bone stronger, it can only repair the damage caused by the collapsing bone.

AIDS

Acquired immunodeficiency syndrome (AIDS) attacks the immune system, preventing it from stopping abnormal growths and infections. AIDS can make you tired and feverish, but the disease itself doesn't generally cause pain. The infections and the cancers that accompany the disease create pain, so you need to check the appropriate chapter for the type of pain you're having.

Up to 98 percent of AIDS patients lose weight as their body tries to fight the disease, so good nutrition is essential. Foods high in protein, carbohydrates, and other nutrients can give the body the energy it needs to protect itself. Nutritional supplements, such as Ensure, help deliver nutrition, and should be taken between meals, not in place of meals.

CHAPTER 11

ALTERNATIVE AMMUNITION: PAIN CONTROL BEYOND NARCOTICS

Work on,
My medicine, work!

William Shakespeare

ALL DRUGS, WHETHER prescription or nonprescription, alter the body's chemistry, so taking any medicine requires thought and consideration. You need to decide if this drug is going to provide more help than harm. To do that, you have to take an active part in your medical care, asking questions of your health care providers and supplying answers that can help them prescribe the best medication for you.

Pain patients have to be especially alert about their medicines, making certain they don't take too much of a drug, take it the wrong way, or mix it with something they shouldn't. Pain patients might try several different medicines for relief, and they should be careful these various medicines don't interact with each other, or with any medication they are taking for other medical problems. Drugs can block pain, giving relief, but no drug is completely safe, so patients have to be active partners in their care, making certain they understand the medicine, whether it is prescription or nonprescription, and what the doctor hopes to accomplish by prescribing it.

This chapter will give you some information and guidelines about common pain medications, but your library contains entire books dedicated to discussing medicines, both prescription and nonprescription. The *Physician's Desk*

Reference (PDR) is a reference book for doctors and lists both prescription and nonprescription drugs (emphasizing prescription drugs), their possible side effects, and uses. Many other books written for the patient also give more information about any drugs you might be taking. Your librarian will have some suggestions.

Your doctor and your pharmacist can also provide answers for any questions you might have. Never walk away from a doctor's office with a prescription until you understand why you are taking it and what you can expect.

Anyone taking medications, whether prescription or nonprescription, needs to be an active participant in their care. The following list of recommendations should be followed no matter what medicine you are taking, or how well you think you understand it.

Always read the label. Some name brands of nonprescription drugs have more than one kind of medicine, with one type containing acetaminophen, while another is the aspirin form, for example. The label on prescription drugs will tell you how and when to take it and will often offer warnings or cautions.

Follow all of the doctor's and pharmacist's instructions completely. Never assume you know more than they do.

Report all side effects and reactions to your doctor or pharmacist immediately. Side effects and allergic reactions can be dangerous, so don't wait. Allergic reactions often show up as rashes, hives, an increased heart rate, or difficulty breathing, but any unusual symptoms should be reported right away.

Never mix drugs, both prescription and nonprescription, without talking with your doctor or pharmacist. A nonprescription drug you've been taking safely for years may not be safe to take with a new prescription.

Tell all your doctors exactly what medicines you are taking so each one can watch out for possible side effects and interactions. If at all possible, have just one doctor prescribe all your medications.

Tell your doctor about any allergies or sensitivities you might have to drugs or your environment.

Anyone with kidney or liver problems needs to discuss
   any medication, even nonprescription, with their doctor.
Pregnant women, women who are trying to get pregnant, and women who are breast-feeding should
   never take any medication, whether prescription or
   nonprescription, without consulting their doctor.

Patients often wonder about substituting generic drugs
for name brands, and, in general, that is safe. The active
medicine in the generic, both prescription and nonprescription, will be the same as the name brand, but other ingredients, called fillers, can be different. If your doctor
approves, try the generic brand and see if it works as well.
   Chapter 12 on narcotics contains a section titled "Delivering Medication" that tells all the different ways you can
take medicine. Those same methods apply to the drugs in
this chapter also. In the following listings, the drug's generic name is listed first, with common brand names in
parentheses.

NONPRESCRIPTION DRUGS
Acetaminophen

Most people know this drug as Tylenol, but it is sold
under many names and in generic form. A fever reducer
and painkiller, acetaminophen comes in pills, liquid, and as
suppositories. This drug hasn't been proven to reduce inflammation, but it might reduce it somewhat, and it is generally safe and effective in relieving pain. Acetaminophen
doesn't cause as much stomach distress as aspirin and
doesn't keep blood from clotting, like some other nonprescription pain relievers do, so it is often used after surgery
and childbirth.
   Taken in large doses, acetaminophen can cause liver
damage, so never exceed the dose recommended on the
label. This drug has a ceiling effect, which means taking
more than the recommended dose won't produce more pain
relief. Two extra-strength tablets, which contain one gram

of medicine, give the maximum pain-reducing effect.

Acetaminophen is often used in other medications, both nonprescription and prescription, so be sure and read all labels so you don't accidentally take a double dose of this medicine. Allergies to this drug are rare, and it is usually safe to take with other medicines, although you should always check with your doctor or pharmacist.

Aspirin

Aspirin's scientific name is acetylsalicylic acid, and your doctor might also refer to it as ASA. A proven pain and fever reducer, aspirin also reduces swelling, and comes as pills, liquid, and suppositories. As its name implies, though, aspirin is an acid and can upset your digestive system, so always take it with food or take coated tablets. Don't take aspirin if you have a history of ulcers or other digestive system problems.

Aspirin is also a blood thinner; it lengthens the time it takes your blood to clot, so it increases the time you bleed before your body repairs the damage. If you've been taking aspirin and cut yourself, you'll probably bleed a little longer before a scab forms. Sometimes this can cause bloody noses or if you already have hemorrhoids, they can bleed more easily. Never take aspirin if you're taking a prescription blood thinner unless your doctor says to, and don't take aspirin with nonsteroidal anti-inflammatory drugs (NSAIDs), because these lengthen clotting time, also. Never take aspirin in the last three months of pregnancy without talking to your doctor. Some patients take baby aspirin daily because it is a blood thinner. Studies have shown that it can prevent some heart attacks and strokes, but check with your doctor before taking it on a daily basis.

Aspirin can change blood sugars in diabetics, and it can cause asthma or make it worse in some patients. High doses might cause ringing in the ears. Don't take aspirin with steroids, some antiseizure medicines (such as valproic acid), or with the chemotherapy drug methotrexate.

Reye's syndrome, a rare but serious disease that destroys the liver, can be caused in children and teenagers if they take aspirin while they have a virus, such as the flu or chicken pox. If children under eighteen years of age are ill, it's best to give them acetaminophen or NSAIDs and avoid aspirin.

Aspirin, like acetaminophen, is often used in combination with other medicines, both prescription and nonprescription, so always read labels to see exactly what you're taking. Aspirin has a ceiling effect, so taking more than two extra-strength tablets won't give any more relief.

Nonsteroidal Anti-inflammatories (NSAIDs)

Nonsteroidal anti-inflammatories (NSAIDs) are one of the newest drugs in the pain war. Like aspirin, NSAIDs relieve pain and reduce swelling, and some reduce fever. Not all of the more than twenty NSAIDs are chemically related, but they are grouped together because they produce the same effect. Ibuprofen was the first prescription NSAID, and then became the first one approved for over-the-counter (OTC) use. All the NSAIDs began as prescription drugs, but when tests proved they were safe, many were then approved for nonprescription use. These drugs are available in pill and liquid form, and some are available as suppositories. Like aspirin and acetaminophen, NSAIDs are sometimes combined with other drugs, such as in cold medicines.

Because they are different, some might work for your pain, while others won't work as well. You need to try a new NSAID for two weeks to see if it works because it can take that long for it to reduce swelling. Never take more than the dose recommended on the label unless you check with your doctor.

Like aspirin, NSAIDs thin the blood, so never take them with aspirin or prescription blood thinners. They can cause nosebleeds, and if you already have hemorrhoids, they might bleed more easily. Even a small bump on the head

can cause you to bleed inside your skull when you're taking
these drugs. They can change a diabetic's blood sugars and
can induce asthma or make it worse. NSAIDs can cause
diarrhea, and in some rare cases, constipation.

NSAIDs can also upset your stomach, so always take
them with food. Don't drink alcohol while taking NSAIDs
because it can increase your chances of getting an upset
stomach. If the NSAIDs are working for your pain but up-
setting your stomach, your doctor might be able to prescribe misoprostol (Cytotec), which has been proven to
prevent gastric ulcers.

These drugs can also interact with many antibiotics, so
always check with your doctor before taking NSAIDs. You
might have to switch the type of NSAID you're taking, or
you might have to try another pain reliever. Don't take
them with some of the antiseizure medicines, such as valproic acid and phenytoin. NSAIDs shouldn't be taken with
steroids unless recommended by your doctor.

Some common nonprescription NSAIDs include ibuprofen (Advil, Motrin IB, Nuprin, Midol IB, and Medipren),
naproxyn (Aleve and Naprosyn), and ketoprofen (Orudis).
New ones are constantly being tested, so check with your
pharmacist or doctor to see which one they recommend for
you.

Other Nonprescription Drugs

A visit to any drugstore can overwhelm you with a choice
of pain relievers, including liniments and creams. Many
will contain at least one of the drugs listed above, so always
read the label to see exactly what you're taking. Some pills
are designed just for back pain, while others are marketed
as headache relievers, and you just have to experiment to
see which one works best for your type of pain. Always
follow instructions on the package and check with your
doctor or pharmacist to make sure you don't combine drugs
that might not be safe.

Liniments and creams can help with some muscle and nerve pain near the skin. Again, you just have to experiment with these to see if they work for you. Creams containing capsaicin, which is derived from chili peppers, need to be handled with extra care. Wash your hands thoroughly after applying the cream, or use rubber gloves. This cream can sting a bit, but if it hurts too much, soak a paper towel in milk and place it on the site. Never apply the cream near sensitive skin, such as the face, or near blisters, rashes, or other breaks in the skin. Capsaicin has to be consistently used for several days to affect painful nerves.

The only steroid available without a prescription is hydrocortisone cream. It reduces swelling and itching, but doesn't relieve pain. It is often used for rashes, bug bites and stings, and mild hives. Some doctors use it for shingles, while others think it might make the outbreak worse.

PRESCRIPTION DRUGS
Acetaminophen

Prescription acetaminophen comes in the same strengths it does over the counter, but if you have health insurance that only pays for prescription drugs, your doctor can prescribe it, saving you money. Many prescription medicines combine acetaminophen with other drugs, so ask your doctor or pharmacist to tell you what's in your medication so you'll know exactly what you're taking.

Aspirin

Like acetaminophen, prescription aspirin is the same strength as its nonprescription form, but is prescribed so patients can pay for it through their health insurance. It comes in pills, liquid, creams, and suppositories. It is often combined with other drugs in prescription medications, so make sure you understand exactly what you are taking.

Nonsteroidal Anti-inflammatories (NSAIDs)

There are more than twenty prescription NSAIDs, primarily newer drugs and stronger versions of those sold over the counter. Read the section on NSAIDS under Nonprescription Drugs for more information on these drugs.

Doctors prescribe NSAIDs for mild to moderate pain, both short and long term. These drugs are available primarily as pills, but in some cases they can be injected intramuscularly or intravenously. Some are available as suppositories.

Some of the newer NSAIDs don't have to be taken as often as the older ones, and some don't cause as much stomach upset, while others may have fewer side effects. Diflunisal, for example, tends to have fewer side effects than other NSAIDs and doesn't thin the blood. Check with your doctor and pharmacist to make certain you understand all the potential side effects and interactions of the NSAID they prescribe. The NSAID phenylbutazone, prescribed primarily for arthritis and gout, can't be prescribed for more than a few weeks because it affects the blood.

Some common prescription NSAIDs include diclofenac (Voltaren), diflunisal (Dolobid), etodolac (Lodine), fenoprofen (Nalfon), flurbiprofen (Froben), ibuprofen (Motrin), indomethacin (Indocin), ketoprofen (Orudis), meclofenamate (Meclomen), mefenamic acid (Ponstel), nabumetone (Relafen), naproxen (Naprosyn), oxaprozin (Daypro), phenylbutazone (Cotylbutazone), piroxicam (Feldene), sulindac (Clinoril), and tolmetin (Tolectin). NSAIDs available in Canada but not in the U.S. include floctafenine (Idarac), tenoxicam (Mobiflex), and tiaprofenic acid (Surgam). Etodolac, meclofenamate, and oxaprozin are not available in Canada.

Muscle Relaxants

This group of drugs does just what its name says: they relax muscles that have tightened, causing pain. These drugs work in the brain to relax spasms, muscles that have contracted because of injury or illness, giving them a chance to loosen, breaking the cycle of pain and giving the muscle a chance to heal itself. They do not relieve pain, though, so patients often are told to also take a pain reliever. Muscle relaxants are often prescribed for myofascial pain, back pain, strains, sprains, or other types of muscle pain.

Muscle relaxants can cause blurred vision, sleepiness, drowsiness, light-headedness, a dry mouth, and, rarely, nausea. Most side effects from this group of drugs disappear after you take them for a while.

These drugs can exaggerate the effect of tricyclic antidepressants and can increase the drowsiness and lethargy sometimes caused by other depressants, such as narcotics and alcohol.

Some common muscle relaxants available in pill form are carisoprodol (Soma), chlorphenesin carbamate (Maolate), chlorzoxazone (Paraflex, Parafon), metaxalone (Skelaxin), methocarbamol (Robaxin), orphenadrine (Norflex), and cyclobenzaprine (Flexeril).

Baclofen (Lioresal) is available as a pill and for use in intrathecal pumps. Sometimes prescribed for RSD, it can cause muscle weakness. Baclofen in the pumps can cause respiratory depression, which means you might not breathe as fast as you should. Always taper off this drug and don't suddenly stop taking it because it might cause muscle spasms and confusion.

Diazepam (Valium) helps with sleep, is an antiseizure medicine, and an antianxiety medicine, as well as a muscle relaxant. This drug has a high potential for abuse, and many other drugs are now available, so it usually isn't the first drug a doctor will prescribe for pain. Never drink alcohol with this drug because both depress the respiratory system. Diazepam can make you drowsy and unable to concentrate.

Steroids

Steroids slow the body's immune system response, which reduces swelling, itching, and any allergic reaction. By reducing swelling, steroids get to the source of pain, helping it where it begins, but they are not pain relievers. Often used for cancer pain, rheumatoid arthritis, and autoimmune diseases such as lupus, steroids have many side effects that must be weighed against their potential for helping before using them in the long term.

Because steroids slow down the body's immune system, taking them increases your risk of infection because the body can't attack viruses and bacteria as quickly or as well when you take steroids. When taking steroids, always tell your doctor as soon as you develop any signs or symptoms of illness or infection, including a cough or fever. Also, because steroids suppress your immune system, keeping your body from making its own steroids, never suddenly quit taking them. Always taper the dose if you want to stop, giving your body time to begin making its own.

Steroids can upset your stomach, so always take them with food. They can also cause nervousness, trouble sleeping, increased appetite, and fluid retention, so your face and body may become puffy. Taking steroids for more than two weeks can increase your chances for developing cataracts, diabetes, osteoporosis, and unwanted face and body hair.

Steroids can alter the effects of blood thinners and insulin, so consult with your doctor before taking them. Steroids also interact with heart and antiseizure medicines. Never get a vaccine made from a live virus when on steroids, and it's a good idea not to get any vaccines while on steroids because you won't get the immune response necessary for the vaccine to work.

Some common steroids available in pill form are cortisone, prednisone, methylprednisolone, dexamethasone, and prednisolone.

Tricyclic Antidepressants

Developed to help depressed patients, tricyclic antidepressants (TCAs) also help with nerve pain. These drugs alter signals in the brain, but scientists aren't sure just why they help with pain. It may be they somehow interrupt or change pain signals. Antidepressants aren't considered pain relievers, but when combined with proven pain relievers, they often help calm nerve pain. Do not take them for pain unless your doctor prescribes them for that purpose, and don't take them for other pains you may develop.

This group of antidepressants also restores normal sleep patterns. Sleep is essential for healing, especially with muscles, so these drugs give the body a chance to sleep and relax, allowing sore muscles a chance to get better.

Tricyclic antidepressants are one of the older drugs for depression, and studies show they do help with pain. Scientists are experimenting with some of the newer antidepressants, and they may help with pain, but there are no studies to prove it. Doctors sometimes prescribe the antidepressants trazodone (Desyrel) and maprotiline (Ludiomil) for pain, even though they aren't tricyclics.

All antidepressants work in the brain, with each one working a little bit differently. They depress the central nervous system, slowing the brain and body and changing the way nerves conduct signals. You shouldn't take any drug, prescription or nonprescription, with tricyclic antidepressants without first checking with your doctor or pharmacist.

Common side effects of tricyclic antidepressants include a dry mouth, dizziness, drowsiness, constipation, increased appetite, nausea, weight gain, and headaches. Never abruptly stop taking these drugs and talk with your doctor about how to taper off these medications.

Because they depress the nervous system, tricyclic antidepressants can make the effects of other depressants worse. Don't take alcohol, barbiturates, narcotics, or benzodiazepines without first talking with your doctor.

Don't take nonprescription cold and flu medicines, including nose sprays, with tricyclic antidepressants without checking with your doctor or pharmacist. These drugs can interact, causing high blood pressure.

Cimetidine (Tagamet), a medicine for upset stomachs, can increase the effects of these antidepressants, so that you might have to reduce the amount of tricyclic you take. Any medicine that also causes a dry mouth, such as antihistamines, can make the effect worse in patients taking antidepressants.

Tricyclic antidepressants can interact with blood pressure and heart medications, preventing them from working. The blood thinner warfarin (Coumadin) can also interact with antidepressants, so you may not need to take as much of the warfarin.

Most tricyclic antidepressants are taken orally, but some are also available for intravenous use. Some common ones are amitriptyline (Elavil, Endep), amoxapine (Asendin), clomipramine (Anafranil), desipramine (Norpramin, Pertofrane), doxepin (Sinequan), imipramine (Tipramine, Tofranil), nortriptyline (Pamelor, Aventyl), protriptyline (Vivactil), and trimipramine (Surmontil).

Antiseizure Medicines

Doctors have known for decades that antiseizure medicines help relieve pain, but they don't know why. These drugs alter signals in the brain, and it could be that they somehow change pain signals, too. Used primarily for nerve pain, antiseizure medications are sometimes prescribed by themselves but often are combined with other known pain relievers.

These drugs must be taken on a regular schedule to be effective. By keeping a steady amount of antiseizure medicine in the bloodstream, they can consistently suppress pain signals. Only use this medicine for pain when prescribed by your doctor. Do not take it for other aches and pains. All antiseizure medicines can have serious side effects, so only take them under the supervision of your doctor.

Carbamazepine (Tegretol) is available in both pill and liquid form. It can cause dizziness, sleepiness, nausea, vomiting, blurred vision, balance problems, and confusion. This drug can also cause a potentially fatal blood problem, so your doctor must constantly monitor your blood while you are taking it. Carbamazepine interacts with more than 100 other drugs, including some that might be used for pain control, so never take anything else, including nonprescription medications, without checking with your doctor.

Gabapentin (Neurontin) is the newest antiseizure medicine used for pain, and it doesn't have some of the dangerous side effects of older medications. Available as a pill, gabapentin can cause sleepiness, dizziness, tiredness, and sometimes imbalance.

Phenytoin (Dilantin) is available as a pill, liquid, intravenously, and as a shot in the muscle. It can cause psychological changes, slurred speech, trembling, constipation, nausea, vomiting, dizziness, sleepiness, gum problems, and other serious side effects. Your doctor will monitor your blood levels while you take this drug because if you take too much, you have an increased risk of developing side effects. Like carbamazepine, phenytoin interacts with many drugs, so never take anything else, including nonprescription medicines, with it without first checking with your doctor.

Valproic acid (Depakene) can potentially cause liver damage, so your doctor will monitor your blood levels while you are on this drug. Available as pills and liquid, valproic acid can cause abdominal pain, decreased appetite, nausea, vomiting, diarrhea, and weight gain. It can interact with many medications, including aspirin, so always check with your doctor before taking anything else with it.

Headache Medications

Oxygen is used to stop cluster headaches after they begin. It is breathed through a mask, usually for fifteen or twenty minutes. The oxygen prescribed by your doctor is 100 percent oxygen, compared with the 21 percent oxygen content of air, so you're getting about five times the amount. Oxygen is highly flammable, so never smoke while breathing it or get near any kind of open flame. Oxygen doesn't cause fires, but it can feed one that gets near it. Oxygen can make you feel better, which is why you sometimes see athletes breathing it on the sidelines, but follow your doctor's instructions completely when using it. Too much oxygen at this high concentration for too long can cause lung damage.

Ergot alkaloids are used for cluster and migraine headaches, and they prevent blood vessels from dilating or constricting too much, helping to keep normal pressure in the brain. All of this group of drugs have serious side effects and interact with many other drugs, so always follow the doctor's instructions completely. If you have any vascular or heart problems, be sure and tell your doctor before taking any of these drugs. Ergot alkaloids also interact with nicotine, which can cause the vessels to constrict more than they should. They can cause nausea, vomiting, numbness or tingling of the fingers and toes, sleepiness, a dry mouth, dizziness, and diarrhea.

Ergotamine tartrate (Medihaler Ergotamine, Ergomar, Ergostat, Cafergot, Wigraine, Bellergal-S) is often combined with other drugs, such as caffeine, aspirin, or acetaminophen, and is available as a suppository, pill, and as an inhaler that you spray into your mouth. Using the inhaler form can make asthma worse. You can become physically dependent on this medicine, so it is generally only given for short periods.

Dihydroergotamine mesylate (DHE 45) comes only as a shot and doesn't seem to cause physical dependency. It can cause heartbeat abnormalities, though, and the first time you get a shot will probably be in an emergency room or a hospital so a doctor can monitor your heartbeat.

Methysergide maleate (Sansert) is used to prevent migraine and cluster headaches, but it is generally prescribed only when other medicines haven't worked. It can't be used continuously because it can cause scar tissue to form around internal organs, so patients have to take breaks from it.

Beta blockers were originally developed to help with high blood pressure. These drugs slow the heart rate, keeping pressure down in the brain. Used to prevent migraines and some tension headaches, not all beta blockers work for headaches. These drugs can cause nausea, diarrhea, light-headedness, trouble sleeping, they can worsen asthma, and make you feel tired when you take higher doses. You must learn to monitor your heart rate when taking these drugs, and your doctor will teach you how to do this. Beta blockers come as pills, and some common ones include propran-olol (Inderal), atenolol (Tenormin), metoprolol (Lopressor), nadolol (Corgard), and timolol (Blocadren).

Calcium channel blockers were developed to help control high blood pressure. These drugs relax the muscles around blood vessels, so blood can move more normally. They can be used to prevent migraines, cluster headaches, and doctors report they help with some tension headaches. They can make you feel tired, dizzy, light-headed, nauseous, and they can cause headaches. They interact with heart medicines, but always check with your doctor before taking any other medications with these. Some common calcium channel blockers prescribed for headaches include diltiazem (Cardizem), nimodipine (Nimotop), nifedipine (Adalat, Procardia), and verapamil (Calan, Isoptin).

Combination medications are used for both migraine and tension headaches. These drugs are usually taken as pills after a headache begins to try to stop it. They contain a pain reliever and a mild sleep aid, which allows you to relax. There's generally not enough sleep aid to make you sleep, but they can make you drowsy. Combination medicines are addicting, and you become physically dependent on them if you take them regularly, so you have to be extremely careful and follow your doctor's instructions completely. Most of the time, though, you aren't taking these drugs on a daily basis. If you are taking them regularly, never stop suddenly, but taper the dose according to your doctor's instructions. Some common combination medicines prescribed for headaches include Esgic, Fioricet, Fiorinal, Phrenilin, and Phrenilin Forte.

Sumatriptan (Imitrex) breaks a migraine, and up to 75 percent of patients report it stops their headache. Available as a shot and a pill, sumatriptan should be taken as soon as you feel a migraine beginning, although it will work even during a migraine. If your doctor thinks it's safe, you can give yourself injections of this drug at home with a special syringe. It works on the blood vessels in the brain, relieving the pressure of the migraine. Usually, the first time you try this drug will be in a doctor's office because it can cause chest pain and a short, temporary increase in blood pressure. If you have heart disease or uncontrolled high blood pressure, make sure your doctor knows that before you try sumatriptan. This drug can cause dizziness, tingling in the hands and feet, a warm or hot sensation, tightness in the chest, and discomfort at the site of the shot.

New Pain Drugs

Tramadol (Ultram) works as well as narcotics for some patients, although it isn't chemically related to them. Studies show it is as effective as narcotics for many types of pain without the dangers of physical dependence and addiction. Scientists aren't exactly sure how it works, but it seems to operate in the brain.

Tramadol is available as pills and can cause nausea, constipation, headaches, sleepiness, and dizziness. It interacts with the antiseizure medicine carbamazepine, which makes tramadol not work as well.

Mexiletine (Mexitil) was originally developed for patients with abnormal heart rhythms, but it seems to help with pain, especially nerve pain. It's chemically related to lidocaine, a local anesthetic, but can be taken as a pill.

Mexiletine can cause nausea, vomiting, dizziness, confusion, and imbalance. The smaller the dose, the less chance of side effects. Occasionally, this drug can cause liver and blood problems. It interacts with the antiseizure drug phenytoin, and you may have to take more mexiletine to get the same effect. It also interacts with the tuberculosis drug rifampin.

CHAPTER 12
NARCOTICS

But, for the unquiet heart and brain,
A use in measured language lies;
The sad mechanic exercise,
Like dull narcotics, numbing pain.

Alfred, Lord Tennyson

THE WORD NARCOTICS evokes fear and awe in the human mind, linking it with junkies, drug wars, opium dens, and addiction. It is certainly a class of drugs in the pain arsenal that must be handled with caution and care, but for the chronic pain patient, narcotics, either in the short or long term, might give relief when everything else fails. But these are drugs of last resort, and they should only be prescribed when the pain arsenal is exhausted. For multidisciplinary pain centers, the goal is to get patients off narcotics if at all possible and keep them off, because these drugs have so many side effects.

The Greeks wrote about narcotics in the third century B.C., and Arabian physicians are believed to have introduced it into the Orient, where it was used mainly to control dysentery. Opium, the dried juice from the poppy plant, was the original narcotic, and it wasn't until 1806 that a chemist distilled morphine from the juice. He named it for Morpheus, the Greek god of dreams. Later, other scientists learned to make codeine, which is ten times less powerful than morphine, and other drugs from opium.

Morphine and opium were legal in the United States until the early 1900s, and they were often used in the patent medicines of the time. Morphine was widely used by wounded soldiers during the Civil War and was also used in diet aids because it can suppress the appetite. It wasn't until 1928 that medical journals described it as addictive.

Today, the term opioid refers to a class of drugs that have the same properties as opium. In the United States, these drugs, including morphine, are made synthetically in a lab, and not from the poppy plant. Morphine and its sister drugs do relieve pain, but they aren't perfect, so scientists are still creating new pain relievers that mimic the result but have fewer side effects.

Heroin is made in the step before opium becomes morphine, and when you take it, the body breaks it down into morphine. In Europe, heroin is still used for pain control, but in the United States, doctors prefer synthetic morphine.

Morphine has become the base narcotic, meaning other narcotics are rated on whether they are stronger or weaker than morphine. Morphine is an excellent pain reliever and can help almost everyone with pain, but some people can't tolerate the side effects, while others are allergic to it, so scientists have developed alternative narcotics as well as nonnarcotic pain relievers.

Narcotics are classified as natural, semisynthetic, and synthetic, depending on how they were created. Even though it is now made in laboratories, morphine is considered a natural narcotic because it was originally derived from the poppy plant. Meperidine (Demerol) is a semisynthetic because scientists created it by starting with morphine and adding new chemicals. Synthetic narcotics, such as fentanyl, have no relation to the opium plant, but mimic the effects of drugs that do come from it.

Narcotics work by imitating the body's own painkillers, endorphins and enkephalins. The body releases these natural chemicals when the brain gives the signal, but humans can learn to train the mind to make more of them through psychological training that teaches relaxation techniques and biofeedback. The body can't make enough to handle extreme pain, so doctors substitute narcotics or other pain relievers.

Doctors use narcotics for pain relief, as antidiarrhea medicine, and to suppress coughs. They are best for organ, muscle, and bone pain, but not as good for nerve pain because they require much higher doses to calm nerve pain than they do for other types, which increases the risk of side effects.

These drugs are excellent for pain after an operation, for cancer pain, and for short-term pain. They are sometimes used for chronic pain but should only be prescribed after other drugs and techniques have failed. There's no written criteria for when and how to use narcotics, although in some states it is still illegal to prescribe these drugs for more than ninety days, a law which is frequently ignored.

SIDE EFFECTS

Narcotics are not the first drug of choice because of their many side effects. Always discuss any side effects with your doctor, because he may be able to help you with the symptoms. Some of the side effects are dangerous, so never mix narcotics with any other drug without talking it over with your doctor, and always follow your doctor's instructions.

Narcotics are depressants, which means they slow down the body, including the brain. You respond slower when on narcotics. For example, if you accidentally stick your finger in a fire, it takes your body longer to pull it out. Patients can't think as well or as quickly when taking narcotics, and they often don't think the same way as when they are off the drug.

All narcotics depress the respiratory system, which regulates your breathing. You don't breathe as fast when taking narcotics, which means your body can't get rid of carbon dioxide, a waste product of breathing, as quickly. If you're running and have been taking narcotics, you don't breathe as fast as you normally would, and carbon dioxide levels begin to build in the brain. If enough carbon dioxide builds up, it knocks out the body's drive to breathe. Usually, when someone dies from overdosing on narcotics, it's because they've taken a dose high enough to prevent the body from remembering to breathe.

The body becomes physically dependent on narcotics. This doesn't mean you are addicted, which is psychological, but your body becomes used to having narcotics and depends on them. Physical dependence usually occurs after taking the drug for two to four weeks, but it won't happen at all if you're only taking one pill a day. It also won't happen if the dose is varied, if you take a half a pill one day, then two the next, and then none the following day, for example.

If you are taking narcotics for chronic pain, never stop taking the drug without tapering off on your dose and checking with your doctor. Withdrawal symptoms include nausea and vomiting, restlessness, nervousness, diarrhea, abdominal cramping, muscle aches and pains, sweating, shivering, shaking, and clammy skin. Narcotic withdrawal makes you feel terrible, but it is very rarely life threatening. If you have stomach flu, or some other reason you can't continue taking your narcotics by mouth, then your doctor can give you rectal suppositories or a patch that releases narcotics slowly through the skin.

Almost everyone gets constipated on narcotics because they slow down the bowels. Eating a diet high in produce and whole grains will help with this, and you might need a fiber supplement, which you can buy without a prescription. Nonprescription stool softeners help some patients, and your doctor can prescribe drugs for the constipation if none of the above methods work. Enemas are fine as long as they are only used once in a while. If you need enemas regularly, then talk to your doctor.

Narcotics stimulate the nausea center in the body, sometimes causing nausea and vomiting, which usually goes away after a few days of taking the medication. If you begin feeling nauseous, lie down and take it easy until the feeling goes away. Stick to clear liquids (which are liquids you can see through, like apple juice, sports drinks, and soft drinks) until your stomach feels better, then move up to other liquids, and when you're feeling better, switch to solid food. Call your doctor if you aren't able to keep down your medication. In general, over-the-counter antacids won't work for this nausea because the problem is in the brain, not the stomach. Sometimes, doctors will give you prescription antinausea drugs to help you until the feeling passes.

If you feel dizzy or light-headed, lie down and take it easy for awhile. This common side effect will usually pass after taking the medication for a few days. Doctors don't usually give any medicines for this side effect, but just wait for it to go away.

Drowsiness is another side effect that usually wears off after a few days. Cancer patients, who might have to take long-term narcotics, are sometimes given amphetamines (which speed up the body) to help with the sleepiness, but these drugs have many side effects, too, so doctors don't usually prescribe them for other patients who take narcotics. A small amount of caffeine might help get you through this drowsy phase.

Narcotics sometimes cause personality changes and can make you feel less aggressive and less emotional. They affect concentration, making it more difficult to focus on what you're doing, and it can give you a false sense of well-being. Most of these symptoms usually go away after a few days.

Some narcotics patients get a dry mouth from the medication, which doesn't usually go away over time. If this occurs, be sure to see your dentist, because this condition can cause dental problems and he can give you some medication to help with the symptoms.

Other side effects include depression of the sex drive, a loss of appetite, bad dreams, headaches, and difficulty urinating. Be sure to discuss these side effects with your doctor so he can suggest treatment.

Narcotics have some very rare side effects, too. They include agitation, tremors, seizures, uncoordinated muscle movements, stiff muscles, short-lasting hallucinations, disorientation, insomnia, visual disturbances, increased pressure in the brain, anorexia, throat closing off, alterations in taste, flushing of the face, increased or decreased heart rate, palpitations, fainting, decreased or increased blood pressure, skin rashes, and numbness and tingling.

INTERACTIONS WITH OTHER DRUGS

Because narcotics depress breathing, it is very important
not to take anything else that also slows down the respiratory system. That's why you must never drink any alcohol with narcotics, because alcohol is also a depressant and
the combination can be lethal. Prescription barbiturates and
benzodiazepines (such as Valium) are also very dangerous
to take with narcotics, so if you are seeing more than one
doctor, be sure and tell them all the medicines you're taking
from the other doctors.

Some nonprescription medicines also depress the respiratory system, and you need to check with your doctor before taking them. These include antihistamines, sleep aids
(but not melatonin), and cold remedies.

Narcotics can interact with lots of medicines, so always
check with your doctor before taking anything else while
on narcotics. Some other drug interactions are listed below.
The generic name is listed first, with common brand names
listed in parentheses.

- The antiseizure medicine carbamazepine
  (Tegretol) with the narcotic propoxyphene
  increases levels of carbamazepine in the
  blood to possibly dangerous levels.
- Monoamine oxidase (MAO) inhibitors (Nar-
  dil) can cause depression and blood pressure
  so high that it can burst vessels in the brain.
- Meperidine (Demerol) can make other narcotics stronger, so the narcotics may need to
  be cut back.
- Tricyclic antidepressants can be taken with
  narcotics, but the side effects of the antidepressants, such as dry mouth and sleepiness,
  might be increased.
- Rifampin, an antituberculosis drug, shouldn't
  be taken with methadone because it decreases
  the effect of the methadone.

♦ Zidovudine (AZT), which is an antiviral drug used primarily for AIDS, shouldn't be taken with morphine because morphine increases the strength of zidovudine, increasing the chance of side effects.

ADDICTION

There are many definitions of addiction, but most tend to center around psychological dependency on a drug. Addiction is the misuse of a medication, taking it for an effect other than the one the doctor intended, and it can occur with many prescription and nonprescription drugs. Addicts tend to abuse almost anything and everything, looking for a different effect. They will even abuse nonprescription drugs, like cold remedies and pain relievers, mixing them to see what happens.

People in pain want their life back; they want the pain to stop. They aren't looking to get high or to experiment with drugs; they simply want to take enough of a medication to stop the pain. In one study of 10,000 burn patients, none became addicted to their painkillers, and in another study of more than 11,000 patients who took narcotics for pain after an operation, only four became addicted.

Chronic pain patients have so much pain that their body can't make enough of the natural painkillers, endorphins and enkephalins, to take care of the pain. Narcotics fill this gap, latching onto the body's pain receptors and calming them so they don't send pain signals to the brain. When you are in pain, narcotics send most or all of their medicine to these pain receptors, not leaving any, or very few, to excite other areas of the brain that give the feeling of being high.

Sometimes patients will experience a sense of well-being for the first few days of taking narcotics, but this does not mean you are addicted. This feeling is simply a side effect of the medicine.

Only a tiny percentage of chronic pain patients taking narcotics ever become addicted. Patients and doctors need to be aware of the possibility of that happening, but most patients who truly need these drugs can take them without worrying about becoming psychologically addicted.

PRESCRIBING NARCOTICS

The Drug Enforcement Administration (DEA) monitors both legal and illegal drug use in this country, and in 1970 developed a schedule that breaks drugs down into five groups. Schedule 1 consists of drugs that have a high potential for abuse and almost no medical use, including heroin, hallucinogens (such as LSD), and marijuana.

Narcotics fall into the next three groups, Schedules 2, 3, and 4, classified according to what the DEA sees as their potential danger. Drugs in Schedule 2, which include morphine, meperidine, and codeine, are considered drugs that have a high potential for abuse because they can cause psychological and physical dependence.

Schedule 2 drugs can only be given to patients with a written prescription and can't be called in over the phone except in emergencies. An emergency might be a hospice patient with cancer who suddenly needs more morphine over the weekend. It isn't an emergency if you run out of pills over the weekend because you forgot to go in and get another prescription. Schedule 2 drugs also can't be refilled without another written prescription, so it's always a good idea to keep careful track of your medication and get another prescription when you have about a week's worth of pills left.

Medicines in Schedules 3, 4, and 5 can usually be refilled and can be called in over the phone. The DEA's classifications can seem confusing, even to doctors. Codeine, for example, in its pure form is a Schedule 2 drug, while codeine combined with acetaminophen falls into Schedule 3. Propoxyphene (Darvon) is equal in strength to codeine, but is in Schedule 4.

All this makes a difference to the chronic pain patient

because regulations affect how doctors prescribe medicine. In some states, for example, doctors are required to fill out three copies of a Schedule 2 prescription, with one copy sent to the state board of medical examiners, one to the pharmacy, and one kept in the office. Studies show that when states switch to triplicate copy prescriptions, the number of prescriptions for drugs in Schedule 2 drops and those for Schedule 3 drugs rise. The number of prescriptions for Schedule 3 drugs rise even higher than the number that were for Schedule 2 because patients now need more of the medicine to get the same relief they did from a Schedule 2 drug.

Each state has a board of medical examiners that oversees doctors and can suspend or take away their license. The doctors sitting on these boards review all claims of malpractice and misbehavior against the state's doctors, policing their profession and hopefully weeding out or punishing those who pose a threat to the public. According to surveys, 40 percent of doctors sitting on these boards don't believe narcotics use for chronic pain patients is ever warranted, despite evidence in medical literature that proves otherwise.

Some doctors feel it is easier to not prescribe Schedule 2 narcotics than to be scrutinized by the board. Not because they've done anything wrong, but because decisions made by these boards are based on its members' personal opinions. There are no written guidelines for how or when to give narcotics, so board members must rely on what they think is best.

Add that to the fact that some states still have laws on the books that make it illegal to prescribe narcotics for more than ninety days, and you can see why some doctors simply won't prescribe narcotics on a long-term basis. Narcotics are a drug of last resort and should never be prescribed unless all other options have failed, but for some chronic pain patients, they are the only hope left.

The fear of addiction also prevents some doctors from prescribing narcotics, despite recent studies that show pain patients almost never become addicted. Some won't give them to patients after surgery, afraid even a few days of these drugs will lead to addiction, while others refuse to give them to patients dying of cancer.

Potential legal problems also prevent some doctors from prescribing narcotics. Pain patients who get relief from narcotics tend to be more active than they were when they were in pain, and resume their normal lifestyle. Doctors and pharmacists warn them not to drive or operate heavy machinery while on narcotics, but both are potential targets of lawsuits if the patient does decide to drive and has an accident.

Potential side effects pose another hurdle when doctors decide whether a patient might need narcotics. These are dangerous drugs that should never be handed out lightly, and all possible side effects and dangers must be weighed before a doctor decides if a patient really needs to use these drugs. Whether or not to try narcotics for pain patients must be done on a case-by-case basis, with doctors balancing the dangers to themselves and their patients before ever considering the use of these drugs.

USING NARCOTICS TO TREAT PAIN

Drug companies constantly experiment to improve narcotics to eliminate as many side effects as possible and to increase the painkilling effects of the drugs. This has led to drugs that have no relation to the opium poppy but that deliver at least some of its results.

One of the latest developments is drugs that last longer than the usual three or four hours per pill, giving a steadier dose of the medicine. Most pills deliver a peak dose, then taper off, and it's this peak that addicts want. Patients in pain don't want the peak, they want a steady dose that delivers a constant level of medicine so their pain is controlled most of the time.

These new drugs, called sustained release medicines, only have to be taken twice a day, and they keep the levels of the drug in the bloodstream at an even dose so the pain relief stays constant. Both morphine and oxycodone come in these longer-lasting forms, but they can cost more than $100 per month. Side effects and physical dependence stay the same with these sustained release drugs, but they keep the patient more comfortable for a longer period of time.

Keeping to a regular medication schedule helps give the same effect when taking the shorter-acting narcotics by keeping levels in the bloodstream as even as possible. Keeping on schedule also helps prevent pain, and studies show that patients who do that end up taking less medication than those who are more erratic about their doses. You don't want to wait until the pain is too much because you'll end up taking more medicine and it won't be as effective as if you'd kept on schedule.

Not everyone needs a steady dose, though, especially if they have the kind of pain that comes and goes. You need to talk with your doctor to determine which method works best for you. Sometimes, other painkillers might work instead of the narcotics. One ninety-year-old patient found taking acetaminophen at bedtime kept the pain down during the night, eliminating a dose of narcotics. Always check with your doctor, though, before experimenting.

Because of the side effects of narcotics, most doctors will prescribe the mildest narcotic that will help with the pain. Milder narcotics tend to have fewer side effects and have less physical dependence than their stronger cousins.

METHODS OF DELIVERING MEDICATION

Narcotics can be administered several different ways. The doctor will decide which form of the narcotic is best for the specific medication and for the individual patient. The most common way to take medication is orally, in pill form or as a liquid. Swallowing a pill or a liquid is portable and easy, something a patient can do on their own. Because pills and liquids have to be absorbed in the stomach, how much of the medicine is used by the body sometimes varies from individual to individual. The body has to process oral medicines through the digestive system, which means you need a higher dose of the medication than if you were given a shot or if it was delivered directly into your veins. Never crush or break up a pill or mix it with a liquid unless you clear it with your doctor first. Some medicines, especially those designed to last twelve hours, might be absorbed differently or they might lose some of their strength if they are broken up before they are swallowed.

Spraying medication directly onto the nasal passages bypasses the stomach, so absorption is more consistent. Some drugs are changed by stomach acid and can't be taken as a pill, so they might be given this way. Nasal sprays are easy and portable, so the patient can take them when and where they are needed.

Transdermal means *through the skin,* and delivering medicine through a patch on the skin helps maintain a consistent level in the body, without the highs and lows of medicine gradually being used up and then being replaced. Patches are usually placed on the trunk of the body where the medicine can be absorbed best. Running a fever or being cold affects the way the medication is absorbed, with cold slowing down the delivery and a fever speeding it up.

Some people have a reaction to the adhesive on the patch and can't wear one, while very hairy skin interferes with the body's ability to absorb the medicine. Never cut or puncture a patch because that will affect the way the medicine is absorbed.

Medicine delivered through the rectum in suppository form is absorbed faster than it is in the stomach, and the medicine is released much more consistently when it is inserted properly. This method is especially helpful for patients who are nauseated or who can't swallow pills.

Only insert the medicine one to three inches into the rectum, and always remove the wrapper before using the suppository. If the suppository has gotten warm and is soft, you can place it in the refrigerator for a few minutes to regain its shape.

Subcutaneous means *under the skin,* and this method uses a needle to deliver medicine under the skin where it can be absorbed without having to travel through the digestive system. Medicine can be given as individual shots or through a small pump about the size of a pack of cigarettes that delivers a steady dose through a needle implanted under the skin.

The pump is usually given to cancer patients. There's no pain once the needle is inserted, and the patient can lead a normal life while wearing the pump. There is a slight risk of infection where the needle pierces the skin, and the needle can accidentally be pulled out, but this is rare.

Intramuscularly means *in the muscle,* with the medicine being delivered through a needle into the muscle as a shot. This method gives very fast pain relief and the medicine is absorbed predictably through the muscle. It is painful, though, and there's a risk of damage if the needle hits a nerve. This method is not used as much as it once was because there are newer, better ways to deliver medicine.

Intravenous means *in the vein,* and the medicine is given through a shot or an IV tube directly into the bloodstream. This method gives almost immediate relief and is often used for pain after surgery and for cancer pain. The medicine can be given through almost any vein, whether it is in the arm, neck, hands, or feet. This method can be used at home if a permanent catheter is installed in the vein so the patient or the home health care professional can place the needle in the catheter and inject the medication.

Intrathecal and epidural pumps are used most often for pain after surgery or for chronic pain. They are discussed more fully in chapter 13.

TYPES OF NARCOTICS

Narcotics come in a wide range of strengths and uses. The following is a list of the more common ones prescribed for chronic pain.

- ◆ **Buprenorphine** is usually given for pain after surgery. This drug shouldn't be used with other narcotics because it can make them not work as well. Sometimes prescribed as Buprenex, it is usually given as a shot that lasts about six hours.
- ◆ **Codeine** comes in both liquid and pill form and lasts about three to four hours per dose. It is often combined with aspirin or acetaminophen but can be prescribed by itself. By itself, codeine is listed as a Schedule 2 drug, but not when it is mixed with another medicine. Codeine is used for both short-term and long-term pain control and is also used in prescription cough medicines.
- ◆ **Dihydrocodeine** is sometimes prescribed under the trade name DHC. This drug is used only when combined with aspirin and caffeine because scientists discovered it gives more effective pain control when mixed. Milder than morphine but stronger than codeine, it comes as a pill that is usually taken every four hours. Be careful not to take additional aspirin when taking this drug, because you could get too much in your bloodstream.
- ◆ **Fentanyl** is a Schedule 2 drug that is sometimes prescribed under the trade names Sublimaze and Duragesic. It was originally developed for pain control during surgery. It is still used for that, but today comes in transdermal patches where a steady dose can be absorbed through the skin. It is also used in epidural and intrathecal pumps. Fentanyl lasts only a short time, and if it were given in pill form, it would have to be taken every half hour to hour. Drug companies have also developed a lollipop containing fentanyl for young children to suck on right before sur-

gery, and this method is also being used in cancer patients with nausea.

♦ **Hydrocodone** is also often combined with aspirin or acetaminophen to make it more effective. It is sometimes prescribed under the names Vicodin, Lortab, Darvocet, Zydone, and Anexia, and comes in both pill and liquid form. This narcotic seems to have fewer side effects than some others and is usually taken every four hours, although a long-acting form is being developed. Be sure to stick to the recommended dosage, and don't take aspirin or acetaminophen with hydrocodone to avoid taking too much of those drugs.

♦ **Hydromorphone** is a Schedule 2 drug that is stronger than morphine and is usually reserved for severe pain. It is taken every two to four hours and is sometimes prescribed under the name Dilaudid. Hydromorphone can be given as a pill, as a suppository, in an IV, or in shot form, and is also used in epidural and intrathecal pumps.

♦ **Levorphanol** lasts longer in the body and only has to be taken two or three times a day, but it can build up in the blood, causing respiratory depression. Marketed under the name Levo-Dromoran, it comes as a pill, but can also be given in shot form.

♦ **Meperidine**, also known as Demerol, is a Schedule 2 drug that is generally used for pain after surgery and for short term pain, but it is also used in intrathecal and epidural pumps for chronic pain. If you are taking it in pill form, never exceed 400 milligrams a day because meperidine can accumulate in the body and can cause seizures, agitation, and muscle spasms. This drug can also be given in shots or through an IV.

◆ **Methadone** was originally developed to help heroin addicts avoid withdrawal symptoms, but doctors discovered this Schedule 2 drug is also a pain reliever. It is often prescribed generically, but is also sold under the name Dolophine. Methadone only has to be taken twice a day and comes in pill, liquid, and shot form, and can also be given through an IV.

◆ **Morphine** is the grandfather of all narcotics and the others are judged according to whether they are as effective for pain control. Morphine comes under many names. Used for cancer pain, pain following surgery, as well as both short- and long-term pain, morphine comes in pills, suppositories, liquid, as shots, in IV form, and in intrathecal and epidural pumps. Longer-lasting forms, often prescribed under the names MS Contin or Kadian, can last up to twelve hours. Other forms of morphine usually last two to four hours.

◆ **Oxycodone** is a Schedule 2 drug that is often prescribed for pain after surgery as well as for chronic pain. Sometimes prescribed under the names Percodan, Percocet, Tylox, and Roxicet, it is usually mixed with aspirin or acetaminophen, so ask your doctor which one your medicine has so you don't take more than you should. Pills containing oxycodone are usually taken every four hours, although a longer-lasting form called Oxycontin is usually only taken every twelve hours.

◆ **Oxymorphone** is used primarily for pain after surgery. This Schedule 2 drug can also be used if the patient is having problems taking morphine. Given as suppositories, shots, and in IV form, oxymorphone lasts usually four to six hours and is sometimes prescribed as Numorphan. This drug has the advantage of not suppressing coughs like some other narcotics, and doctors often want patients to breathe deeply and cough after surgery to avoid pneumonia.

- ♦**Propoxyphene**, like some other narcotics, can accumulate in the body, so usually doctors prescribe less than 500 milligrams a day. Never exceed the dose recommended by your doctor. Propoxyphene, which is sometimes prescribed as Darvon, can cause dark urine and pale bowel movements as well as jaundice (yellowing of the skin). It is available in pill and liquid form and is usually taken every four hours.

MIXED NARCOTICS

Scientists have developed a new group of narcotics designed to be less addictive, calling them mixed narcotics. It is very important never to combine any of these drugs with pure narcotics because it can cause withdrawal symptoms and make the drugs less effective. These drugs are rarely used for cancer pain because they can't be mixed with other narcotics, but you can take them with aspirin, acetaminophen, and NSAIDs.

If you are taking narcotics, it is very important that all your doctors know exactly what medications you are taking so they don't prescribe a pure narcotic with a mixed one, and so they don't give you a mixed narcotic for pain after surgery if you are already taking another narcotic.

- ♦**Buprenorphine** is used primarily for pain following surgery. This mixed narcotic is sometimes sold under the trade name Buprenex. It is given in shot and IV form.

 ◆ **Butorphanol**, sometimes prescribed as Sta-
   dol, can make you sleepy and cause hallucinations. It is given as a nasal spray for
   headaches and in shot and IV form for other
   types of chronic pain.
 ◆ **Nalbuphine** is sometimes prescribed as Nu-
   bain. This drug doesn't cause as much respiratory depression as other narcotics, and is
   usually used for pain following surgery and
   is given in shots or in IV form.
 ◆ **Pentazocine** can be given in shot or pill
   form for chronic pain and usually lasts three
   to four hours. Sometimes prescribed as Tal-
   win, it can cause hallucinations.

Narcotics should never be the first drug of choice for
chronic pain, and whenever possible, they should be
avoided because of their side effects. But for some patients,
they are the only thing that works. Narcotics can be used
safely, but the patient must work closely with the doctor
and follow all instructions carefully to avoid problems and
complications.

CHAPTER 13
THE BIG GUNS: NEW TECHNOLOGIES

Yes, in the old days that was so, but we have changed all that, and we now practice medicine by a completely new method.

Molière

A S INTEREST AND awareness of pain control grows, more research dollars and time are devoted to helping patients. Some of the results have been brand-new technologies and methods, such as intrathecal pumps, but some are new uses for established medical technologies, such as harnessing the powers of radio frequencies.

Most patients recover with a minimum of technical devices, but for those who don't respond to more conservative methods, this new technology offers hope where once there was none. Some of these are so new that not all health care providers may be aware of them and their potential benefits.

Technology is usually combined with medicines and hands-on techniques, such as chiropractic care, physical therapy, massage, or acupuncture, because doctors have learned that the combination of therapies works better. Supervision and education are essential when using these new devices because patients need to understand how and why they work in order for them to be safe and effective. These new methods require minor surgery and anesthesia and are not to be handed out indiscriminately, but in the right circumstances, they can truly be lifesaving devices.

It's important that patients understand these devices and methods, also, so they can ask appropriate questions and can understand how and when their health care provider might use them. Potential patients should always ask how many of these technical procedures the doctor has performed and what is his or her individual success rate. You might want to talk with other patients who've had these procedures to see what they think of them.

CRYOANALGESIA

For thousands of years, humans have known that cold compresses relieve pain. In the early 1800s, doctors discovered spraying ethyl chloride cooled the skin and numbed the area for surgery. Toward the end of World War I, doctors sprayed ethyl chloride on injuries to ease pain, but found it didn't work in all cases. By the 1960s, scientists developed safer, more exact techniques using cold gases, such as carbon dioxide and nitrous oxide, that kill specific nerves and ease pain.

Today, doctors use a probe with a tip of at least –28°F to kill the painful nerve. The nerve eventually regenerates, but it takes anywhere from days to years to grow back. Patients with cancer pain, shingles, pain from injuries, rib pain, and extremity pain might benefit from this procedure.

If the patient has a very specific area or nerve causing pain, and if other techniques like medications, physical therapy, relaxation therapy, biofeedback, and nerve blocks haven't worked, the pain specialist might consider cryoanalgesia. Arthritis pain, for example, would not benefit from this technique because the pain is spread over too large an area. The health care professional must be able to identify a specific nerve or nerves causing the pain.

Using local anesthesia, a small incision is made near the troublesome nerve and the cryoprobe inserted. The physician uses X rays to guide the probe, and when the correct location of the nerve is identified, the probe is cooled to kill it. Positioning the probe takes the most time because the physician must make certain the correct nerve is identified and that the cryoprobe will not harm any nerves that control movement (motor nerves). It takes three or four minutes of cooling to kill the nerve, and for the first few seconds, it's uncomfortable, but then the pain stops. Cryoanalgesia may not completely eradicate the pain, but in up to 80 percent of cases, it reduces it significantly.

Cryoanalgesia sounds drastic and complicated, but actually the risk of complications is low. The most common complication is frostbite of the skin where the probe is inserted. Even if the doctor accidentally freezes a motor nerve, they almost always regenerate. The bad news is doctors can't predict how long the pain relief lasts. Sometimes it works only for a few days, while some patients get relief for years.

The cost of cryoanalgesia ranges from several hundred dollars up to $1,000, depending on the location of the nerve and how many nerves are killed. It's usually done in a hospital or surgery center because it requires an X ray machine, but is an outpatient procedure. Medicare covers this technique as do most insurance plans.

RADIOFREQUENCY

Radiofrequency jumps to the other end of the spectrum, using heat, instead of cold, to kill painful nerves. High frequency energy waves create heat up to 190°F on the tip of an electrical probe to kill nerves that feel pain but don't control movement. Like cryoanalgesia, it is always done under X ray, and the pain must come from a specific nerve or nerves for this technique to succeed.

Originally tried in the 1950s, radiofrequency technology couldn't control the temperature at the tip of the probe, sometimes damaging normal nerves and tissue surrounding the painful area. In the 1980s, technology developed a probe that controlled temperature and the burn area, increasing its use in recent years. But this refined technique is too new to have long-term studies, so statistics on its effectiveness are still sketchy. One study did show that for specific types of low back pain, radiofrequency was 66 percent effective.

Like its cousin cryoanalgesia, doctors can't predict how long it will take for the nerve to regenerate. Some patients get relief for years, while for others, it only lasts a few days. The patient will actually experience more pain after radiofrequency, as the burned area heals, usually lasting from one to four weeks.

The jury is still out on exactly where and when radiofrequency should be used, but studies are beginning to show that cryoanalgesia will probably work better for damaged nerves close to the skin, while radiofrequency may be best for nerves deep within the body. Radiofrequency may replace some surgeries, such as sympathectomies (cutting sympathetic nerves), since it is a less invasive technique.

Radiofrequency is usually done in a hospital or surgery center because it must be done under X ray. Costs vary from several hundred dollars to $1,000, depending on where and how many nerves are killed. This procedure is covered by Medicare and most insurance companies.

SPINAL CORD STIMULATORS

Spinal cord stimulators (SCS) have roots as far back as 2600 B.C., when acupuncture techniques were first described. By manipulating the acupuncture needles, a faint electrical current was generated to stop the cycle of pain. Benjamin Franklin took the idea a step farther in the 1700s and used a generator to pass electrical current over painful areas. Even early in this century, scientists experimented with rats and discovered that stimulating the spinal cord using small amounts of electricity affected other parts of the body, such as the skin or toes. So the idea of using electricity to stop pain is not new, but modern technology refined the concept into a practical method for controlling pain.

In 1967, researchers published the first clinical trials showing that patients could get pain relief by electrically stimulating the spinal cord. Initially, spinal cord stimulators required major surgery and often had complications, including infection, equipment failure, and unreliability. By the 1980s, technology and techniques improved to make spinal cord stimulation a reliable and safe procedure, with a success rate of 70 to 75 percent. But it is still a highly technical procedure and should only be performed by physicians who are specially trained and are part of a multidisciplinary pain center. Before considering a spinal cord stimulator, the patient should always ask the physician how many stimulators he or she has implanted and what is his success rate. You may also want to talk to other patients who have stimulators to get the patient's perspective on what it's like to have the procedure and how it affects their life.

Stimulators work best with chronic pain that has stayed pretty much the same over a long period of time. The intensity of the pain can fluctuate, but the location should not. Like most technology, stimulators are one of the last lines of defense in the pain arsenal because they reside in the body and are expensive. In most cases, more conservative measures will take care of the pain. SCSs can be removed with no ill effect for the patient, so they are often tried before techniques that kill nerves, like cryoanalgesia and radiofrequency.

Conservative measures didn't work with Yolanda, a petite twenty-five-year-old office administrator, who broke her left ankle as she slid into home base during a weekend softball game. Using plates and screws, doctors pieced her ankle back together that night and she went home to recover. Three months later, doctors went back in to remove the plates and screws because the bones had healed and Yolanda was ready to resume her busy schedule.

Her recovery from the second surgery was more painful than from the first because she'd developed reflex sympathetic dystrophy (RSD), a condition that restricts blood flow to the injured area, causing intense pain. It hurt just to wear socks or shoes, and her weekend athletics were put on hold because she found it difficult to even walk. Doctors took

X rays to see if the ankle had healed properly and could find nothing wrong.

Physical therapy gave a little relief as did a TENS unit (transcutaneous electrical nerve stimulator), which uses electricity on the surface of the skin to block the pain signal, but she still couldn't walk without what she described as burning, aching, stabbing, shooting, sharp, and prickly pain. It hurt just to touch the foot, and it turned cold and blue.

By now, Yolanda was taking many medications, including narcotics, to help with the pain, which allowed her to work but do little else. After four months with no improvement, her surgeon sent her to an anesthesiologist, who diagnosed RSD and gave her a series of nerve blocks and specialized physical therapy. She began seeing a psychologist who taught her biofeedback and relaxation techniques, which didn't help. The nerve blocks completely removed the pain, but only for a few hours. She tried different medications, but nothing gave long-term relief.

Eventually, Yolanda began taking antidepressants because she was so discouraged about her pain and only wanted to live a normal life again. She traveled to a larger city to get a second opinion and doctors there tried destroying the nerve through radiofrequency. But instead of getting better, the pain spread.

A year and a half after her collision with home plate, Yolanda's surgeon sent her to a multidisciplinary pain center where the doctor confirmed the RSD diagnosis and tried some new medications that had just been released for RSD treatment. Like everything else, these didn't work, and the doctor suggested a spinal cord stimulator. Her psychologist agreed that she was a good candidate, and she underwent the surgery. Yolanda immediately got 90 percent pain relief, and was able to quit all her medications and resumed all her previous activities, except for softball, which she'd decided just wasn't her game.

Modern spinal cord stimulators use electricity to block the pain signal to the brain. The patient doesn't receive a shock, because the current is high enough to interrupt the pain signal, but not high enough to hurt the patient. Many say it feels like a warm whirlpool over the area where they used to have pain.

Implanting a spinal cord stimulator involves two procedures. In the first one, a wire with four to eight electrodes at the end is placed in the epidural space (the area just outside the spinal canal). The electricity crosses the dura (the covering around the spinal canal) and blocks the pain signal in the dorsal column. The dorsal column houses the sensory and pain fibers of the spine. Until recently, patients with pain in more than one area, such as in the arms and legs, couldn't be helped by stimulators, but now doctors are able to use two sets of electrodes to control pain in both areas.

The patient is lightly sedated during the procedure, sleepy enough to be comfortable, but awake enough to talk to the physician, so he or she can tell the doctor when the electrode is in the correct spot. It's in the correct spot when the patient feels a light, tingling sensation over the painful areas.

The most important part of the procedure is making certain the electrode is in the correct position. Once the electrode is in place, the doctor can only move it through another surgery. The patient then usually goes home for a week and tries out the stimulator to make certain it works properly. Many doctors will not implant the permanent device unless the patient comes back a week later and tells them it has made a difference in their lives. Placing a foreign object in the body is too big a risk if the results are only mediocre, not to mention the cost of the permanent stimulator.

Some patients have good results for the first forty-eight hours after placing the temporary stimulator, but then it quits giving them the relief they expect. After a week, if the patient is not delighted, the device is removed in a quick outpatient procedure. If the results make it worthwhile, the patient then undergoes the second procedure of installing a permanent stimulator. One manufacturer offers an external and an internal battery, while the other offers just an external battery. Manufacturers are also working on a rechargeable internal battery and hope to have it on the market soon.

If the doctor uses the first brand, the patient has a choice as to whether they want a battery about the size of a silver dollar and a quarter-inch thick implanted where they can't see or feel it, or whether they want an external battery, which is about the size of a cigarette pack and clips onto an article of clothing or in a pocket. Few patients choose the external battery, because most simply don't want to deal with the outside pack.

Patients with two sets of electrodes must use the external battery because of the amount of electricity needed. The external unit uses a nine-volt battery that has to be replaced every day or up to every week, depending on the amount of energy the patient needs. The patient turns the unit on and off and regulates the power to get the required effect. Sometimes patients develop sensitivities, such as a rash, to the adhesives used with it. Any time the patient takes a bath, showers, or swims, the battery must be removed. It won't kill you to get it wet, but it could give a nasty shock.

The internal unit's battery lasts from three to seven years, depending, again, on how much power the patient needs. Changing the battery requires about an hour of outpatient surgery under local anesthesia. The patient turns the unit on and off using a small magnet. A hand-held device is used to regulate the power, and the patient can adjust it, depending on what works. The patient can swim, bathe, and shower with this unit on or off because everything is under the skin.

In the first phase, the electrode costs about $1,500. There's also a hospital fee, and fees for the physician and anesthesia. The internal battery in the second phase costs about $7,000, but if the patient prefers the external battery supply, the cost is about $5,000. As with the first part, there are also hospital, anesthesia, and physician fees. Most insurance policies cover the cost, and Medicare does, also. Medicare HMOs have a review process and might deny coverage, but they must offer the benefit.

EPIDURAL AND INTRATHECAL NARCOTICS

One of the latest technologies, epidural and intrathecal (sometimes also called intraspinal) narcotics combine established methods with new ideas. Narcotics are appropriate treatment for certain patients, but when given by mouth or by shot, they affect the entire body, which results in undesirable side effects, including, but not limited to, constipation, drowsiness, breathing difficulties, and nausea. In the early 1980s, researchers wondered why doctors should treat the entire body with narcotics when the pain was located in specific areas.

Originally, scientists developed this technique to help patients who had surgery. By giving these patients narcotics by mouth or injection, it made them too sleepy and unable to help with their own recovery. Doctors wanted them up and walking as soon as possible after surgery, but the combination of pain and narcotics kept them in bed. Lying in bed can lead to blood clots in the legs, pneumonia, pulmonary emboli (blood clots in the lungs), and bed sores, so health care providers want patients up and moving as soon as possible after surgery.

Researchers decided to try delivering narcotics intrathecally and epidurally by pumps to block the postoperative pain but keep the patient awake and alert. *Intrathecal* refers to the space housing the spinal cord (the spinal canal), while *epidural* refers to the space next to the spinal canal. Narcotics in both spaces should work equally well, but each have advantages and disadvantages. This technique was not only effective for surgery patients but has benefits for chronic pain patients, especially cancer patients and those with uncontrollable muscle spasms. Epidurals have also become a mainstay for women delivering babies, allowing them to give birth more comfortably and safely.

Intrathecal narcotics deliver medicine directly to the spinal cord, which is the most efficient method for getting

narcotics where they are needed. Picture the spinal cord as
string cheese, where individual nerves are packed together
into a solid string. Where your ribs stop, it begins to fray,
as the individual nerves head on their own path to the hips,
legs, and feet. This is where narcotics can be administered
with the least risk. When the cord is a solid structure, a
needle could damage it, or even sever it, but where the cord
frays, medicine can be injected into the spinal space more
safely.

The epidural space runs from the base of the skull to the
tailbone. It isn't even a real space, but the area between the
ligamenta flavum (ligaments that support the spinal vertebrae) and the dura (the sack surrounding the spinal canal),
where the physician inserts a specialized needle to create a
space between the two tissues. A catheter is then inserted
into the space, delivering narcotics or other pain relief medicines to where they're needed. Intrathecal injections are
almost always done below the rib cage, but epidurals can
be given anywhere the space runs.

Once a catheter is established in either the epidural or
the intrathecal space, it is usually attached to a pump that
delivers medicine continuously or whenever the patient
feels he or she needs it. Epidural pumps are about the size
of a portable cassette player, and hang on a belt or fanny
pack. The patient controls the amount of medication by
pushing a button, giving themselves a boost whenever they
need it. Intrathecal pumps are about the size of a hockey
puck and are usually surgically implanted underneath the
skin on the abdomen, with the catheter following just under
the skin around to the intrathecal space. Some are programmed to dispense specific amounts of medication at a
certain time, while others continuously deliver a set amount
of medicine. One cancer patient, for example, knew her
priest visited every day at 2 P.M., and she wanted to be able
to get out of bed and receive communion, so her pump gave
her a boost of medication at 1:30 each afternoon. The epidural catheter and pump usually cost about $1,500 to
$2,000.

Drugs used regularly in the pumps include fentanyl and

hydromorphone, both narcotics. Local anesthetics that are approved for spinal anesthesia but not for pain control are also placed in the pumps. Because the medicine is delivered directly where it is needed, the risk of addiction to the narcotics is almost zero. The body will become dependent on the medications, just as it can be dependent on high blood pressure medicine, so there would be some physical symptoms if the medication were to be stopped too quickly, but the patient is not addicted. Stopping the medication abruptly can cause sweating, rapid heartbeat, nausea, pain, and muscle cramping, almost like a really bad case of the flu. It is not life-threatening, just uncomfortable.

There are advantages and disadvantages to both epidural and intrathecal pumps. The advantages of an epidural include lower initial cost than the intrathecal pump. Only a one-inch incision is needed in the back to install the epidural, with a small hole in the patient's side where the other end of the catheter comes out to attach to the pump. More varieties of medicines can safely be placed in the epidural space than the intrathecal space.

One of the disadvantages for the epidural is that the pump is always on the outside of the body, making it more awkward to take a bath or a shower, and the external unit may interfere with some daily activities, such as sleeping. Over time, the epidural is more expensive than the intrathecal because it uses much more medicine; doses have to be increased to get the same effect as placing them in the intrathecal space. If the pump will be used more than three months, it is more cost effective to use an intrathecal pump instead of an epidural. Because the end of the catheter comes out of the body, an epidural requires extra care and is more prone to infection.

The intrathecal pump is more convenient for patients because it rests completely under the skin, and because less medicine is needed; it only has to be refilled every two weeks to ninety days, compared with possibly every few days for an epidural. Refilling an intrathecal pump usually requires a trip to the doctor's office, while an epidural can be refilled by home health care professionals.

For short-term pain, doctors sometimes place the catheter in the intrathecal space and attach it to a pump that stays on the outside of the skin. This is much less expensive than installing a permanent pump because you don't have to buy it, but pay a daily rental fee. There's an increased chance of infection because the pump isn't planted under the skin.

Rick, seventy, spent his retirement traveling with his wife to Las Vegas, Texas, and other parts of the West. One day, he began vomiting blood at home and his wife took him to the emergency room. Suspecting bleeding in the stomach, surgeons opened him up and discovered cancer throughout his abdomen. They repaired the bleeding stomach, but the cancer had spread too far and too fast to do anything about it.

Doctors placed him on pain medication after the surgery, but as the cancer continued to spread, the increasing doses of medicine made him nauseous and extremely constipated. The pain and the side effects from the medicine prevented him from traveling and enjoying retirement, even though the cancer had not yet slowed him down. His cancer doctor referred him to a multidisciplinary pain center. Because the pain radiated throughout his abdomen, Rick wasn't a good candidate for nerve blocks, so the doctor decided to try epidural narcotics. A temporary epidural brought relief immediately, and a permanent one was installed two days later. Rick resumed traveling with his wife, and although he continued to have complications from the cancer, he was able to do almost everything he wanted.

All patients who are candidates for these methods have tried oral narcotics and possibly intravenous narcotics or narcotics administered by injection, and either they didn't get enough pain relief or the side effects were too harsh. Some suffer severe constipation; others may be too woozy from the oral medication. Estimates range from 5 to 25 percent of cancer patients are candidates for these spinal pumps.

One of the latest uses for these pumps are for patients who have uncontrolled muscle spasms caused by spinal cord injuries or diseases such as multiple sclerosis. In these

patients, a medicine called baclofen is substituted for narcotics. Baclofen is a very strong muscle relaxant and gives
these patients relief from the severe muscle spasms that
sometimes plague them. Most get relief from the oral baclofen, but for those that can't, the pump is another option.
Studies show that by controlling the spasms, patients also
have fewer bedsores and fewer infections.

These pumps aren't used very often for long-term pain
control of other chronic pain patients because of the danger
of infection over the life of the catheter and pump. In terminally ill patients, there is a risk of infection, but the risk
is considered to be less than the benefits of pain control.
The same is true with paralyzed patients. In other chronic
pain patients, the amount of medication needed goes up
over time, which means their pump has to be filled more
often, increasing the risk of infection. If the catheter has to
be removed, it can lead to a chronic spinal headache. The
jury is still out on whether this technique will eventually
be useful for other types of chronic pain as researchers
study its uses and benefits.

These advanced pain control techniques can be expensive, especially the implanted intrathecal pumps. Two types
of these are on the market and one costs about $10,000. It
runs on a battery and delivers the exact amount of drug
when the patient wants or needs it, around the clock. The
other one costs about $5,200, and doesn't use a battery, but
instead uses the principles of physics to deliver medication.
It delivers less exact doses and cannot be programmed for
individual needs.

Patients can travel with both types of pumps. Facilities
to refill and reprogram the programmable pumps exist in
almost every major city in the United States and other in-
dustrialized countries. The pump can be read by a hand-
held computer in the doctor's office that tells what
medication it uses and how much and when. With the non-
programmable ones, whoever is refilling it must check with
the doctor who installed it to find out how much to use and
what medicine it contains.

Both have to be implanted in an operating room, but

frequently can be done on an outpatient basis. Anesthesia, physician fees, and operating room costs are about the same for both types of pumps. Refilling the pumps with medicine costs approximately the same, although the solution for the less expensive pump has to be custom mixed and might cost a bit more. Narcotics cost anywhere from $100 to $300 to fill the pumps, depending on the type of solution used, and they have to be filled anywhere from every two weeks to three months, depending on how much medication the patient needs. Baclofen, for muscle spasms, costs about $600 to fill the pump, but only has to be refilled every three months. In addition to the cost of the medicine, there are office or hospital fees and possible physician fees. Home health care companies can fill these in the patient's home if he or she cannot get to the hospital or doctor's office.

EPIDURALOSCOPY (MYELOSCOPY)

Before CAT scans and MRIs, doctors needed to see inside the spinal column to make a diagnosis. In the 1930s, doctors designed a myeloscope to examine the spine by looking down a tiny tube inserted into the spinal canal while the patient was anesthetized. The technique worked, but it never really caught on, and it disappeared from medical studies until the late 1960s.

As doctors began experimenting with the technique again, they modified the myeloscope, which looked directly at the spinal cord, to an epiduraloscope, a fiber optic scope that is more flexible and smaller, to examine the epidural space (the space between the spinal canal and the ligament that holds the vertebrae together). By looking in the epidural space, they could see nerves leaving the spinal cord, discs, tumors, and scar tissue. The fiber optic scope allows doctors to see conditions missed by MRIs and CAT scans. Epiduraloscopy, also called myeloscopy, is especially effective at identifying small pockets of scar tissue, small herniated discs, and nerve root inflammation, conditions that cause pain, but went undetected before.

This technique and equipment are still being studied and were recently approved by the Food and Drug Administration. Universities around the country are conducting trials to see if epiduraloscopy lives up to its promise, but the technique is only available in a few areas of the country.

The hope is that by identifying these tiny patches of scar tissue or inflammation that can't be seen by current methods, doctors will be able to use the scope to break up the scar tissue, inject medicines, or possibly do surgery through the scope, the way many abdominal operations are now performed. Early reports show this technique holds lots of hope for the chronic pain patient, but careful studies must be completed.

New weapons are constantly being tried in the battle against pain, offering new options for the pain patient and health care providers. As doctors learn more about how pain works, they keep trying new medicines, new technologies, and new knowledge to help their patients. No technique or method works for everyone, but by arming themselves with information, patients can ask the right questions and make certain they are getting the treatment they need.

CHAPTER 14

NAVIGATING THE MINE FIELDS: HOW TO GET THE HELP YOU NEED

You may have to fight a battle more than once to win it.
Margaret Thatcher

GETTING THE RIGHT kind of help may be the biggest challenge faced by chronic pain patients. Pain will not kill you, and is not considered a life-threatening condition, so insurance companies and health maintenance organizations (HMOs) have little incentive to act quickly about your pain. Pain can be expensive to treat, and some insurance companies hope that by delaying treatment, you will become dissatisfied and switch plans.

Recent belt-tightening measures in the health care industry now scrutinize every expenditure, which can keep premium costs down, but can leave pain patients battling for relief. Understanding the industry, and especially your individual policy, is the first step in getting help.

TYPES OF INSURANCE

Indemnity plans were the first forms of health insurance in this country, but they have declined in recent years. These plans allow you to choose your own doctor, hospital, and laboratories, usually paying 80 percent of the fee. You are responsible for the remaining 20 percent, up to a certain amount, and then the insurance plan covers all the costs. There is usually no preauthorization with these plans.

Preferred provider organizations (PPOs) are similar to indemnity plans in that you can use the doctor and facility of your choice, but if you use ones on their preferred list, you have fewer out-of-pocket expenses. These plans might require some preauthorization, especially for surgery.

Health maintenance organizations (HMOs) are the latest trend in health insurance, although they've actually been around for decades. You have a choice of doctors with HMOs, but the doctors must be ones on their list. Your doctor, though, even if he is on their list, may not be able to continue seeing you if you switch to an HMO. Sometimes doctors have a set number of patients that the HMO pays for, and if they are full on that plan, they cannot continue treating you. Be sure and call your doctor to make certain he can take you on that plan before you switch. The hospital and laboratories you get to use are set by the HMO, and almost all procedures and visits to specialists must be preapproved by your primary doctor or a medical committee.

HMOs often pay their doctors a set fee per patient, per month. If a doctor has 500 patients under your HMO, he gets a certain amount of money each month whether he sees one patient that month or all 500. The fee doesn't change, no matter what illness or complications a patient has. In some HMOs, doctors are given bonuses if they don't admit too many patients to the hospital or order too many tests, and in some cases, a doctor is penalized financially if he admits too many. Some HMOs employ their doctors, paying them a salary to see the HMO patients, and these employees often operate under the same financial rules.

Pain patients may have difficulty getting referred to a pain doctor under HMOs, because the pain doctor probably doesn't work under the same financial arrangements as the primary doctor. The pain doctor is usually paid out of a fund for specialists, and it costs the HMO, and possibly the primary doctor, money to send you to a pain clinic.

Any patient with a chronic condition tends to not do as well with HMOs, whether it is chronic pain or some other condition that requires continuous treatment. A recent study showed that 54 percent of chronically ill Medicare patients declined in physical health with HMOs, compared to 28 percent who were treated under indemnity or PPO plans. The study found no statistical difference in patients who didn't have chronic illness.

If your HMO contract covers pain control, then you are entitled to that care. Your HMO may try to stall treatment, hoping you'll get frustrated and take your expensive diagnosis to some other plan. Chronic pain won't kill you, so there's no medical reason for them to hurry and provide treatment. Keep fighting, though, because you've paid for that care.

When they first became popular, HMOs had less expensive premiums than PPOs and indemnity plans, but that is not necessarily the case now. PPOs and indemnity plans tend to have lower overhead than HMOs because they let doctors make treatment decisions and don't depend on a bureaucracy of committees and paperwork before allowing a patient access to treatment. So shop around, and carefully choose an insurance plan that best suits your needs.

KNOW YOUR POLICY

With all three types of plans, you need to know what is and is not covered in your policy, and the limits to what is covered. If you don't understand the policy, call the sales representative and have them explain it to you. Psychological counseling, for example, may not be covered, or it could be limited to a certain number of sessions. The same is true with physical therapy, chiropractic care, and just about anything else. Very few policies cover any alternative or experimental medical procedures.

The technologies and treatments listed in this book are covered by most insurance plans, and you can ask your insurance representative about your coverage. If you are covered, then you are entitled to that treatment. If you are covered by an HMO, ask your doctor if he is bound by a gag rule. Some HMOs restrict doctors from telling you about medical procedures that they don't cover, as if they didn't exist at all. Doctors in PPO and indemnity plans can tell you about treatments not covered by your policy, and give you the choice of paying for it yourself.

MEDICARE

Medicare is divided into two parts: one that covers hospital costs and one that covers doctor expenses and other costs. The cost of medicines, some mental health services, and some nursing home services are not covered by Medicare. As anyone who's dealt with Medicare knows, rules and regulations complicate even the simplest transaction, and administrative costs now exceed all payments made to doctors.

These tangled rules and regulations, though, can benefit the pain patient if you're willing to wade through the extensive review processes established to protect you. Medicare offers excellent pain benefits and covers every technique described in this book. If you have a Medicare HMO, you are entitled to every benefit the government allows for Medicare, but you might have to fight a little harder to get those benefits. Medicare has specific grievance procedures to follow if you think you aren't getting appropriate care, and your local Medicare office or your HMO can get you started. The federal government is currently reviewing these procedures to make certain HMO patients get the care they need.

Medicare HMOs are paid a set fee by the government for each person they enroll. That amount of money doesn't go up or down no matter what problems the patient develops, so the less money the HMO spends on each patient, the more money it will make. The government likes HMOs because its costs stay the same for each patient, but some patients report having trouble getting the type of care they are used to receiving, although their benefits stay the same as they would under any Medicare plan. But patients don't have any extra expenses with these HMOs, because the HMOs take care of all the bills. Like any HMO, you're limited to the doctors and hospitals that are a part of that plan.

Other insurance companies, besides HMOs, are now offering these supplemental policies where they receive a set fee from the government and then you don't pay any additional fees, no matter what services you need. Some of these cover medications, mental health services, and many nursing home services.

Until recently, doctors could set their own fees and bill the patient for whatever Medicare didn't cover. Today, though, participating doctors must accept whatever Medicare pays them. Doctors can choose not to participate in Medicare. Patients who are part of Medicare are billed by the doctor, who is only allowed to charge 5 percent more than the fee set by Medicare, and payment is made directly to the patient.

Medicare has steadily cut back its fees to physicians, so that some doctors are now limiting the number of Medicare patients they will see, while others won't take on any new Medicare patients. For some specialties, doctors are paid fees they charged back in the 1970s or 1980s.

WORKMAN'S COMPENSATION

When you are hurt on the job, workman's compensation handles your treatment, not your regular health insurance policy. Your employer selects the type of workman's compensation coverage, and it can be an indemnity plan, a PPO, or an HMO.

Your employer selects the plan, but he doesn't select the doctors you can use. As long as the doctors are affiliated with the plan, you can use them. Employers sometimes suggest specific doctors for their workman's compensation employees, but you don't have to go to those doctors in most states.

Workman's compensation laws vary from state to state, so you'll have to check with your union or workman's compensation board to find out exactly what benefits are covered. In Texas, for example, workman's compensation only pays benefits for two years, and then you revert to your regular health insurance plan.

In general, workman's compensation offers good pain benefits because they want you to go back to work, and you can't go back to work if you are in pain. All techniques described in this book are generally offered to pain patients, but may not be offered right away. Workman's compensation boards usually have review processes you can use if you think you aren't getting the treatment you are entitled to. You need to know your rights and the rules and policies in your state.

HOSPICE CARE

Hospices provide emotional support, pain control, and medical services for the terminally ill. Staffed by specially trained health care professionals, hospices provide services for both the patient and the family, emphasizing comfort for the patient over life-prolonging procedures. Although many people think of hospices as a place to go to die, they also provide home health care services for the terminally ill who can and want to stay at home.

Hospices do not perform any life-saving techniques like heart transplants or chemotherapy but emphasize keeping the terminally ill patient comfortable while offering emotional and psychological support for the family. If you are in active treatment—receiving radiation therapy, for example—that will stop when you enter a hospice. You will continue taking your regular medication, but no new treatments will be started.

Many hospices are associated with hospitals, but they aren't technically a part of the hospital and have their own staff trained to work with the terminally ill. Sometimes you are required to change doctors when entering a hospice, but that usually doesn't happen.

Once you enter a hospice, your insurance goes directly to the hospice, which now provides your medications and treatment. If your condition improves, you can always switch back to your regular heath insurance. Almost all insurance policies provide for hospice care, but you need a doctor's order to join a hospice; if you are on Medicare, you can always go to a hospice. Medicare doesn't provide for very much home health care or for drugs, but once you enter a hospice, those items are covered. You are never required to join a hospice, but some patients like the fact that the hospice covers medications, home health care, and psychological counseling.

Hospices emphasize pain control and have access to doctors who are specially trained to keep the patient comfortable and alert for as long as possible. The hospice covers all medication and pain control techniques, and the staff is usually trained to deal with pain control methods.

Many think entering hospices means giving up, but what it really means is accepting what is happening to your body. Hospices offer valuable services for the terminally ill and their families and offer support and guidance at this difficult time.

SELECTING A DOCTOR

Not all doctors understand chronic pain management, and some still believe that most pain is caused by psychological problems, so finding an ally in your pain war may take some searching. It is worth the effort, though, to find the right doctor who will lead your charge into the health insurance battlefield.

All insurance plans have a responsibility to the patient to provide adequate care. If you think you aren't getting it, then you should talk to your doctor. Be persistent about getting the care you need, and if you still feel your doctor isn't responding, then ask for a referral to a doctor who might be more knowledgeable about your condition. It is vital, especially if you are in an HMO, to have a primary care doctor who understands that you need pain control. Without the backing of your primary doctor in an HMO, there's almost no way to get treatment. HMOs have medical committees that allow you to appeal decisions made by your doctor, but if he has decided a treatment is not medically necessary, the committee usually agrees. So you may need to switch primary care doctors. You may need to interview other doctors, and you might have to pay for these visits, but it's important to be your own advocate—you have the right to pain management.

Ask your potential primary care doctor if he is board certified in his specialty, and ask what kind of additional training he's had. All doctors, whether they are family practice, internal medicine, or anything else, can become certified by the American Academy for Pain Management in addition to being certified by their specialty. Your primary care doctor doesn't have to be certified in pain management; he simply has to understand that you need treatment for your pain so he can refer you to someone who does have special training if it is needed. If you're looking for a new doctor, ask friends and coworkers who they like. Checking with any support groups you belong to is another good resource for names.

When looking for a doctor, call his office and ask if he treats patients with your condition. Choose a doctor who specializes in your area. Don't limit yourself to a doctor in your neighborhood. Patients often choose a doctor because he's close to home, but it's worth the effort to drive a little farther to get to a doctor who will do you the most good.

The county medical society can give you names of doctors but won't usually give any more information. If you are concerned about your doctor, you can contact the state medical examination board, which can tell you about any disciplinary action against him, such as malpractice and substance abuse.

SELECTING A PAIN CENTER

Anyone can set up an office and call it a pain center, so you have to be careful when choosing one. The term *pain center* doesn't tell you much; it could be someplace that only offers chiropractic care, or only psychological care, or only nerve blocks. All of these are important parts of pain treatment, but usually the best way to fight pain is at a multidisciplinary pain center offering a combination of treatments.

Not everyone needs a multidisciplinary approach for their pain, but chronic pain often resists treatment and needs to be attacked on several fronts. A multidisciplinary pain center should offer a variety of services, including physical therapy, psychological help, manipulation therapy, medical management of medications, and nerve blocks. Not all these treatments need to be offered by the pain center, but the center should coordinate treatment, referring you to whatever services you need, with doctors and nurses at the pain center following up on your care and serving as a command center for your various treatments. Doctors should evaluate your entire problem, taking time to listen to a history of your pain and how it affects you.

Only M.D.'s (medical doctors), dentists, and D.O.'s (doctors of osteopathy) can prescribe medication, so make certain one of those is available. Certain nurses and physician's assistants can prescribe, but they have to be supervised by an M.D. or a D.O.

Pain centers can be a part of a hospital or be run out of a free-standing clinic, but wherever it is, make certain it has a comfortable atmosphere providing you with privacy. It should have its own nurses and staff who are trained in dealing with pain treatment. Ask if they have a brochure detailing the services they provide and the credentials of their professional staff. They should also be willing to offer you a tour of their facility.

Before you select a pain center, check with your insurance plan to find out which ones you can go to, then ask your primary care doctor for recommendations. Also check with friends and members of any support groups you belong to for suggestions.

Call the pain center and ask about the director and his degree. If he's an anesthesiologist, the emphasis might be more toward nerve blocks; if it's a chiropractor, the emphasis might be on manipulation therapy; or if it's a psychologist or psychiatrist, the emphasis might be on psychological help. Whatever the degree, make certain other treatments are available.

As with any health care provider, check the credentials of everyone treating you, from massage therapists to M.D.'s. Are they licensed by the state? What degrees do they hold? If they are M.D.'s, are they board certified? Being board certified doesn't guarantee a good doctor, but it does mean that physician has taken the extra steps and time to meet the board criteria.

Many teaching and university hospitals have pain clinics, often coordinated by anesthesiologists. Some of these clinics are excellent, but you will probably be treated by residents, who are M.D.'s with their degree, but are completing their training. Residents are always supervised by a faculty member, but if you aren't comfortable with being treated by them, you should seek another facility.

Once you've selected a pain center, bring a list of all your medications, any test results, and a list of all the doctors you're seeing. The health care professionals at the pain center need to know exactly what's going on in your medical life so they can begin evaluating your problem and coordinating treatment.

Certain types of pain need prompt attention, such as shingles and early RSD, and if you're having trouble getting in quickly, ask your primary care doctor to see if he can get you an earlier appointment. Pain centers should be able to make room for emergencies, and you want to go to a pain center that is willing to make room for you.

• • •

Pain patients not only have to battle pain, but often they have to fight with the medical community to get the help they need. As with any struggle, you must carefully choose your allies, making certain they understand pain and are willing to fight for your right to return to a better life. There are health care professionals out there who want to help and who understand the multidisciplinary approach to pain, and their numbers are growing. As medicine understands pain more, more pain patients are finding the relief they deserve.

APPENDIX

American Cancer Society
1599 Clifton Road NE, Atlanta, Georgia 30329; (800) ACS-2345
Free booklets and information on support groups.

American Chronic Pain Association
P.O. Box 850, Rocklin, California 95677; (916) 632-0922
Provides support system for those with chronic pain. More than 800 chapters.

Arthritis Foundation
1330 W. Peachtree, Atlanta, Georgia 30309; (800) 283-7800
Information on support groups and pain management.

Hospice Association of America
228 7th Street SE, Washington, D.C. 20003; (202) 546-4759; Web site: http://www.nahc.org
Hospice referrals, patient information.

National Chronic Pain Outreach Association, Inc.
7979 Old Georgetown Road, Suite 100, Bethesda, Maryland 20814-2429; (301) 652-4948

National Headache Foundation
428 W. St. James Place, Second Floor, Chicago, Illinois
60614-2750; (800) 843-2256
Support groups, newsletter, educational materials.

Reflex Sympathetic Dystrophy Syndrome Association
116 Haddon Ave., Suite D, Haddonfield, New Jersey
08033; (609) 858-6553
Information and referral to support groups.

Spondylitis Association of America
P.O. Box 5872, Sherman Oaks, California 91413; (800)
777-8189
Information and support groups.

Trigeminal Neuralgia Association
P.O. Box 340, Barnegat Light, New Jersey 08006; (609)
361-1014, fax, (609) 361-0982
Information and support groups.

GLOSSARY

acupressure—a variation of acupuncture using finger
  pressure instead of needles.
acupuncture—a pain control technique using tiny
  needles to alter electrical impulses in the body.
acute—brief and severe pain, usually occurring early in
  the disease or injury.
anesthesiologist—a doctor who anesthetizes patients;
  some specialize in pain control.
arachnoiditis—a disease where scar tissue and swelling
  wrap around the spinal cord.
arthritis—disease that causes joints to swell and
  deteriorate.
atrophic—the third stage of reflex sympathetic
  dystrophy.
aura—a sensation, such as a strange smell or change in
  vision, that comes before a migraine.
benign—cancer cells that aren't consuming or replacing
  normal cells.
biofeedback—a method of learning to control body
  functions, such as heart rate and breathing, by
  monitoring brain waves, blood pressure, and muscle
  tension.
blood thinners—drugs that slow clotting time; some are
  prescribed to prevent strokes and heart attacks.

bone scan—a medical test for bone abnormalities using a dye and X rays.

breakthrough pain—a sharp rise in pain, usually caused by exertion or movement.

cancer—any abnormal growth in the body.

capsaicin—a cream that helps control pain; made from chili peppers.

carpal tunnel—the sheath that houses the median nerve as it runs through the wrist.

carpal tunnel syndrome—pain caused by scar tissue in the carpal tunnel compressing the median nerve; usually caused by using the same wrist motion over and over.

CAT scan—computerized axial tomography; sometimes also called CT scan.

causalgia—an injury to a major nerve; usually associated with bullets or shrapnel.

ceiling effect—the maximum dose of medication that is helpful; above that dose, the medicine can be harmful and offers no greater pain control.

central pain syndrome—where an injury or illness in the brain causes another part of the body to feel pain.

cerebral spinal fluid—the liquid that surrounds and protects the brain and spinal cord.

cervical epidural—medicine placed in the epidural space of the cervical spine.

cervical spine—the top seven vertebrae of the spine.

chemotherapy—a method of cancer treatment where drugs are used to try to kill the cancer cells.

chronic—pain that lasts longer than it is supposed to, usually more than six weeks.

complex regional pain syndrome—another name for RSD.

compression fracture—spinal vertebrae that break from normal usage because disease has weakened them.

computerized axial tomography—a specialized X ray showing cross sections of the body; especially good for viewing organs and other soft tissue.

CRPS—complex regional pain syndrome.
CSF—cerebral spinal fluid.
disc—tissue between the vertebrae.
dura mater—the protective membrane covering the brain and spinal cord.
dystrophic—the second stage of reflex sympathetic dystrophy.
electromyogram—a medical test that measures the signal nerves are sending to muscles.
EMG—electromyogram.
epidural space—the area between the ligaments of the spine and the spinal cord; almost all nerves pass through this space.
euphoria—a feeling of well-being, sometimes through medicine.
facet joints—joints between vertebrae that hold the spine in place and allow the spine to move.
failed back syndrome—where a patient continues to have pain even after surgery has corrected the original problem.
fibromyalgia—muscle disease that causes muscles to ache; the cause is unknown.
fusion—spinal surgery where metal rods or bone grafts are inserted, bridging the damaged area.
gag rule—a rule that prevents a doctor from telling patients about treatments not available with their HMO.
half-life—the amount of time it takes half the medication to leave the body.
health maintenance organization—a type of medical insurance plan where the choice of doctors and facilities is limited and where most treatments require preauthorization.
HMO—health maintenance organization.
hospice—a place that supplies care and treatment for the terminally ill and their families.
indemnity plan—a type of health insurance where the company usually pays 80 percent of the cost of

treatment and the patient gets to choose their doctor, hospital, and laboratories.

intramuscular—in the muscle.

intranasal—medicine absorbed through the membranes in the nose.

intrathecal—in the spinal canal.

intravenous—in the vein.

IV—intravenous.

laminectomy—surgery on vertebrae that removes part of the lamina.

lipoma—a benign, fatty tumor.

lumbar epidural—medical procedure where medicine is placed in the lumbar epidural space.

lumbar spine—the lower five vertebrae.

lumbar sympathetic block—local anesthetic is injected into a specific group of nerves in the lumbar region.

lumbosacral—referring to the lower five vertebrae in the spine and sacrum.

magnetic resonance imaging—a specialized X ray using magnetic fields to show detailed images of the inside of the body.

malignant—cancer cells that replace normal tissue.

meniscus—fibrous tissue padding the temporomandibular joint and other joints.

metastasize—when cancer cells spread from the original tumor.

migraine—an extremely painful type of headache, usually on one side of the brain.

motor nerves—nerves that put muscles in motion.

MRI—magnetic resonance imaging.

myofascial pain—muscle pain caused by muscles that stay tensed.

myotherapy—therapy that stretches muscles.

NCV—nerve conduction velocities.

nerve conduction velocities—a medical test measuring how fast a nerve conducts a signal.

neuralgia—pain along an irritated nerve.

neurosurgeon—a surgeon specializing in the nerves, spinal cord, and brain.

nonprescription—medicine that can be bought without a doctor's prescription.

nonspecific back pain—low back pain that doesn't have a cause medical tests can discover; usually muscle or ligament pain caused by a sprain or strain.

nonuseful pain—pain that continues after an injury has healed and serves no useful purpose.

nucleus pulposus—gelatinlike material in spinal discs.

NSAIDs—nonsteroidal anti-inflammatory drugs.

opioid—a class of drugs having the same properties found in opium.

oral—by mouth.

orthopedic surgeon—a surgeon specializing in the skeletal system.

osteomyelitis—an infection of the bone.

osteoporosis—a disease that weakens the bones.

over-the-counter—medicines that can be bought without a prescription.

perimysium—thin layer of connective tissue surrounding individual muscles.

periosteum—tissue surrounding the bones and joints.

peritoneum—protective covering of the organs in the abdomen.

physiotherapy—physical therapy.

placebo—a drug or treatment that is not supposed to have any effect.

PPO—preferred provider organization.

preferred provider organization—a type of health insurance where the patient has fewer out-of-pocket expenses if he uses doctors on the company's list.

radiation treatment—a form of cancer treatment that uses X rays to shrink or kill tumors.

rebound headache—a headache that occurs when a patient takes too much medicine too often; as the medicine wears off, the withdrawal causes another headache.

rectally—medication absorbed through the rectum.

reflex sympathetic dystrophy—a pain syndrome caused by the involuntary sympathetic nervous system constricting blood flow to an injured area.

REM sleep—rapid eye movement sleep, the dream stage.

repetitive stress injury—an injury caused by using the same movement over and over, such as carpal tunnel syndrome.

RSD—reflex sympathetic dystrophy.

RSI—repetitive stress injury.

sacrum—the bone at the bottom of the spine.

scoliosis—congenital disease where the spine curves abnormally.

SCS—spinal cord stimulator.

sensory nerves—nerves that send signals of what the body is feeling.

skin conductance response test—a medical test measuring how the skin conducts electricity.

SMPS—sympathetically maintained pain syndromes.

specific back pain—low back pain that comes from a specific cause, such as a herniated disc or spinal stenosis.

spinal cord stimulator—a pain control device using electrodes in the epidural space to block the pain signal from reaching the brain.

spinal stenosis—where a nerve opening in the spine is too small, causing a nerve or the spinal cord to be pinched.

spinous process—the long bone in a vertebra pointing toward the skin.

stellate ganglia—a group of nerves in the neck that control the sympathetic nervous system on the face, neck, arm, shoulder, and upper chest.

subcutaneous—under the skin, as in injections.

sweat response test—a medical test measuring differences in the amount of sweat.

sympathetically maintained pain syndromes—another name for RSD.

sympathetic nerves—nerves controlling functions humans don't usually control, such as breathing, digestion, and blood flow.

temporomandibular joint—the hinge joint that connects the jaw to the skull.

TENS—transcutaneous electrical nerve stimulator.

therapeutic window—the level of medication where it does the most good with the least side effects.

thermography—a medical test measuring differences in skin temperature.

thoracic epidural—medicine placed in the epidural space of the thoracic spine.

thoracic spine—the middle twelve vertebrae of the spine; the ribs come off these.

thoracic sympathetic blocks—inserting local anesthetic into specific nerve groups in the thoracic region.

tic douloureux—another name for trigeminal neuralgia.

TMJ—temporomandibular joint.

transcutaneous electrical nerve stimulator—a small electrical device, powered by a battery, that transmits electrical impulses to electrodes on the skin; used in pain control.

transdermal—medication absorbed through a patch on the skin.

transverse process—the cross bone of a vertebra that runs at right angles to the spinous process.

trigeminal nerve—a nerve in the face that controls the muscles in the lower jaw and conducts pain signals to most of the face.

trigeminal neuralgia—irritation of the trigeminal nerve in the face causing sharp, one-sided pain.

trigger point—nerve groups in muscles where information is relayed.

tryptophan—an amino acid that helps build nerves.

useful pain—pain that signals something is wrong.

vascular—referring to the blood vessels.

workman's compensation—insurance that handles your health care costs if you are injured on the job; chosen and paid for by your employer.

INDEX

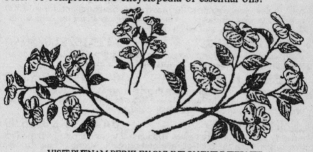